SKILLS PRACTICE MANUAL TO ACCOMPANY

Health Unit
COORDINATING

formerly Unit Secretary

Fifth Edition

Health Unit
COORDINATING

formerly Unit Secretary

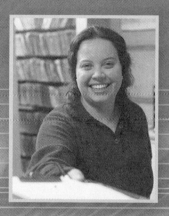
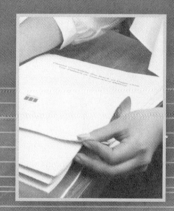
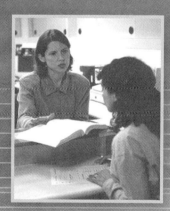

Myrna LaFleur Brooks, RN, BEd, CHUC
Founding President,
National Association of Health Unit Coordinators
Faculty Emeritus, Maricopa County Community College
District
Phoenix, Arizona

Elaine A. Gillingham, AAS, BA, CHUC
Program Director,
Health Unit Coordinator Program
GateWay Community College
Phoenix, Arizona

SAUNDERS
An Imprint of Elsevier

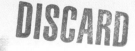

SAUNDERS
An Imprint of Elsevier

11830 Westline Industrial Drive
St. Louis, Missouri 63146

SKILLS PRACTICE MANUAL TO ACCOMPANY HEALTH UNIT COORDINATING   ISBN 0-7216-0099-9
Copyright © 2004, Elsevier (USA). All rights reserved.

NOTICE

Medicine is an ever-changing field. Standard safety precautions must be followed, but as new research and clinical experience broaden our knowledge, changes in treatment and drug therapy may become necessary or appropriate. Readers are advised to check the most current product information provided by the manufacturer of each drug to be administered to verify the recommended dose, the method and duration of administration, and contraindications. It is the responsibility of the licensed prescriber, relying on experience and knowledge of the patient, to determine dosages and the best treatment for each individual patient. Neither the publisher nor the author assumes any liability for any injury and/or damage to persons or property arising from this publication.

Previous editions copyrighted 1998, 1993, 1986, 1979
ISBN: 0-7216-0101-4

Executive Editor: Adrianne Cochran
Developmental Editors: Helaine Tobin, Rose Foltz
Publishing Services Manager: Pat Joiner
Designer: Kathi Gosche

Printed in the United States of America

Last digit is the print number: 9   8   7   6   5   4   3   2   1

PREFACE

The fifth edition of *Skills Practice Manual to Accompany Health Unit Coordinating* reflects and corresponds with the latest changes made in *Health Unit Coordinating,* 5th edition. This edition also includes a CD-ROM, *Practice Activity Software for Transcription of Physicians' Orders.* The health unit coordinating text provides the theory needed to perform the health unit coordinating job, and the skills manual and practice CD-ROM provide hands-on practice in performing the transcription of doctors' orders and other tasks performed by the health unit coordinator.

CHAPTER DESIGN

The chapters correspond with the chapters of *Health Unit Coordinating,* 5th edition. The student learns the theory by reading the chapter and completing the exercises and review questions in the text and then practices the task in this manual. Each activity begins with a list of materials needed and step-by-step instructions to complete the activity. Activities provided in Chapters 10 through 19 may be completed by using the *Practice Activity Software for Transcription of Physicians' Orders* on a computer. When a computer is not available, the activities may be completed by using the requisitions, which are samples of computer screens provided in Appendix B in the back of this manual. Handwritten doctors' orders are included in Appendix A for additional practice in transcription as well as reading handwriting.

CD-ROM

Practice Activity Software for Transcription of Physicians' Orders included in this manual simulates the hospital computer system that students may use for practice when transcribing the printed and handwritten doctors' orders provided. Options provided on the CD for practice include the following:
- Enter orders
- Print a nursing unit census
- Admit a patient
- Transfer a patient
- Discharge a patient
- Research location of patients admitted to the hospital by using "patient inquiry"
- Verify tests ordered by using "order inquiry"
- Cancel an order that has been entered
- Research diagnostic test results by using "laboratory results" or "diagnostic imaging results"
- Locate or create a patient profile
- Enter medications on a patient medication profile
- Order isolation
- Locate a doctor on the doctor's roster

Patient forms may be printed from this CD, making it possible for the student to practice the transcription process at home.

Clinical Evaluation Record

A clinical (on-the-job) evaluation is included in Appendix C of this manual to measure and record the student's performance on the nursing unit. It is divided into seven units; the first six are sequenced according to the increasing degree of knowledge and skill that the student needs to complete the unit. The objectives and corresponding activities will assist the student in mastering each of the tasks required. A rating scale is provided to measure and record the student's performance level.

The Clinical Evaluation Record tells the student, the instructor, and the preceptor exactly what is expected of the student during his or her clinical experience. Use of this record allows the student to pursue mastery of skills and to arrange an evaluation of skills by the instructor or preceptor. The completed appendix becomes a written record of the student's performance in the clinical setting. The appendix may be used by the instructor to assign grades or by the student to obtain employment. As does the rest of this manual, this appendix corresponds with the textbook *Health Unit Coordinating,* 5th edition.

INSTRUCTIONS TO THE STUDENT

HOW TO USE THIS MANUAL

This manual consists of approximately 96 activities that provide practice for the health unit coordinator student to master skills in a simulated hospital setting prior to actual hospital practice. It also includes a clinical evaluation record designed to measure and record the student's on-the-job performance.

The activities in this manual correspond to the content of the same-numbered chapters in the textbook *Health Unit Coordinating,* 5th edition. For best results, read each chapter and complete the exercises and review questions provided in each chapter of *Health Unit Coordinating* prior to performing the activities in this manual.

Chapters

The chapters are numbered and titled to correspond with the chapters of the textbook *Health Unit Coordinating*, 5th edition. The activities match the theory content of each chapter. Textbook chapters that do not require practice are not included in the manual. *There are no activities included for Chapters 1, 2, 3, 5, 6, 9, 20, 22, and 23.*

Each chapter specifies the skill to be practiced, the materials needed to practice the skill, and the steps necessary to perform the skill, with check boxes provided to record completion of each step and of the whole activity. As each activity is completed (preferably after having been repeated until complete accuracy is achieved), either the instructor or the student should write a check in the completion box.

Chapters 4, 7, and 8 include practice in communication skills and in preparing and working with the patients' charts. Chapter 7 includes instruction and practice in preparing a census worksheet (may be printed from CD-ROM), and Chapter 8 includes instruction and practice in assembling a patient's chart (forms may be printed from the CD-ROM).

Chapters 10 through 18 provide practice in transcribing the different categories of doctors' orders. The steps of transcription are repeated in each activity to provide the student with an orderly learning experience and a useful summary for future reference.

Chapters 19 and 21 provide practice in performing health unit coordinating tasks such as admission, preoperative and postoperative procedures, charting of vital signs, and ordering daily diagnostic tests.

Supplies Needed by the Student:
- Computer (when available)
- Black ink pen
- Red ink pen
- Pencil
- Eraser
- Yellow highlighter

Check with your instructor for additional required supplies.

Suggestions to the Student for Maximum Use of Chapters 10 Through 18:

1. At the beginning of each activity, steps may be deleted or added to adapt the procedure to the practice in your area.
2. Record in the spaces below the symbols used to indicate completion of the transcription steps.

   _____ Kardexing
   _____ Ordering (either by computer or requisition)
   _____ Recording the medication on the medication administration record
   _____ Completing a telephone call
   _____ Faxing or sending the pharmacy copy of the physicians' order sheet

3. Record the color(s) of ink to be used for the transcription process.
4. Remove all physicians' orders provided in the activities as directed and place them in the chart binder that you prepared in Chapter 8 to simulate hospital practice.
5. Generic forms and examples of computer ordering screens that may be used as requisitions when computers are not available are provided in Appendix B. You may duplicate these or use forms and requisitions supplied by your instructor to complete the activities.
6. To practice transcribing orders by the computer method, simply use the computer to perform the ordering step by following the instructions included in each activity and the Practice Activity Software for Transcription of Physicians' Orders.
7. Fill in today's date, time, and doctors' names on each practice doctors' order sheet prior to starting the transcription process.
8. Hospitals require that the physicians' orders be faxed to the pharmacy or the pharmacy copy sent. This activity may not be practiced in the classroom.

Appendix A

Appendix A consists of sets of actual doctors' orders. They contain many orders not included in the activities and are written as they might be seen in the actual hospital environment. The sets of orders provide experience in automatic cancellation, renewals, and changes. Practice transcribing the sets of doctors' orders by the computer method using the Practice Activity Software for Transcription of Physicians' Orders or the requisition method by using the requisitions provided and the 10 steps of transcription.

Appendix B

Generic forms and copies of computer ordering screens that may be used as requisitions (when computers are not available) necessary to complete the activities are included in Appendix B. Reproduce as many of each as are needed for each activity.

Appendix C

Appendix C is a Clinical Evaluation Record, designed to measure and record the student's performance in the hospital setting. A rating scale is included to measure and record the student's level of performance. The student should take the Clinical Evaluation Record to the hospital site each day and use it as a guide in obtaining on-the-job experiences and an evaluation rating from his or her preceptor or instructor.

Many of the skills included in this Clinical Evaluation Record are critical; that is, an error in performing them on the job could cause harm to the patient. We hope that by working your way through the activities you will become both competent and confident in your practice, and that you will be ready to accept the full responsibilities of a career in health unit coordinating.

CONTENTS

SECTION 4

Health Unit Coordinator Procedures 175

Orientation to Hospitals, Medical Centers, and Health Care

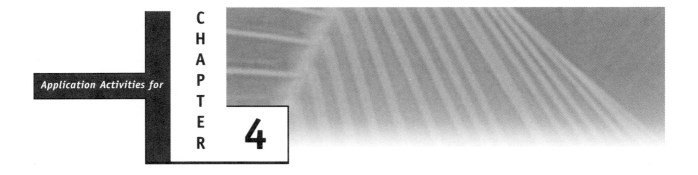

CHAPTER 4

Communication Devices and Their Uses

Activities in this Chapter:

 ## ACTIVITY 4-1

ANSWER THE TELEPHONE

Materials Needed   Telephone
Pen or pencil

Situation

You are a student health unit coordinator on an orthopedic floor, 3 East, at College Hospital.

Directions

Practice answering the telephone using the information in the previous situation. Follow the steps below. Place a check mark (✓) in the box as you complete each step.

Steps for Answering the Telephone

1. Answer the telephone promptly (preferably before third ring). ❑

2. Identify:
   a. the nursing unit ❑
   b. yourself (give your name) ❑
   c. your status ❑

3. Follow correct telephone etiquette by:
   a. speaking into the telephone mouthpiece
   b. giving the caller your undivided attention
   c. being courteous at all times
   d. speaking distinctly and clearly

Place a check mark (✔) in the box below to indicate that you have completed Activity 4–1.

☐ Answer the Telephone   Date: _____

ACTIVITY 4-2

PLACE A TELEPHONE CALLER ON HOLD

Materials Needed   Telephone
                       Pen or pencil

Situation

You receive a call from Sharon Green, the case manager, asking to speak to Harry Rabbett's nurse about his transfer to an extended care facility.

Directions

Practice placing a telephone caller on hold using the information in the previous situation. Follow the steps below. Place a check mark (✔) in the box as you complete each step.

Steps for Placing a Telephone Caller on Hold

1. Follow the steps for answering the telephone as directed in Activity 4–1.   ☐
2. Record the name of the caller, the nature of the call, and which line the call is on: ☐

MESSAGE PAD

Name of the caller: _____

Telephone line number: _____

Message: _____

_____

---

3. Ask permission to place the caller on hold (do not say, "Hang on a minute"); wait for their
   answer.   ☐
4. Depress the hold button.   ☐
5. Notify the nurse of the recorded information, including the telephone line the case worker is on. ☐

Place a check mark (✔) in the box below to indicate that you have completed Activity 4–2.

☐ Place a Telephone Caller on Hold   Date: _____

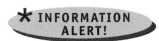

Always return to the person on hold every 30 to 60 seconds to ask if they wish to remain on hold or leave a number for a return call.

ACTIVITY 4-3

RECORD A TELEPHONE MESSAGE

Materials Needed   Telephone
Pen or pencil
Message pad

Situation

Dr. Jan Hurtte telephones your nursing unit. She states: "Notify Judy Jones, RN, that I will be making rounds within an hour to check on Mary Copa's condition."

Directions

Practice recording a telephone message using the information in the previous situation. Follow the steps below. Place a check mark (✓) in the box as you complete each step.

Steps for Recording a Telephone Message

1. Follow the steps for answering the telephone as directed in Activity 4–1. ❏

2. Record the following information on the message pad. ❏

MESSAGE PAD

Who the message is for: _____

The caller's name: _____

The date and time of the call: _____

Message: _____

_____

_____

_____

Telephone number of the caller if a return call is expected: _____

Your name: _____

Place a check mark (✓) in the box below to indicate that you have completed Activity 4–3.

❏ Record Telephone Messages   Date: _____

ACTIVITY 4-4

PLACE A TELEPHONE CALL TO A DOCTOR'S OFFICE

Materials Needed　Telephone
Pen or pencil
Simulated doctors' roster provided by your instructor

Situation

Judy Jones, RN, asks you to place a call to Mary Copa's doctor, Dr. Jan Hurtte, regarding Mary's temperature of 38.2 degrees centigrade. Mary Copa has been diagnosed as having a degenerative arthritic spine.

Directions

Practice placing a telephone call to a doctor's office using the information in the previous situation. Follow the steps below. Place a check mark (✓) in the box as you complete each step.

Steps for Placing a Telephone Call to a Doctor's Office

1. Plan the call by recording the following information on the note pad:　❑

NOTE PAD

Patient's name: _____

Telephone number of the doctor's office: _____

Reason for the call: _____

Person requesting the call: _____

Time call placed: _____

Person spoken to: _____

---

2. Obtain the patient's chart.　❑

3. Select the correct physician using the doctors' roster provided by your instructor by referring to:
　a. the first and last name of the physician　❑
　b. the specialty area　❑

4. Add the telephone number of the doctor's office to the information on the note pad (a time saver in case the telephone line is busy or you have to return the call).　❑

5. Place the call to the doctor's office.　❑

6. Follow the telephone etiquette outlined in Activity 4–1.

7. Give the following information when the telephone is answered:
　a. your name　❑
　b. your status　❑
　c. the name of the hospital　❑
　d. the name of the nursing unit　❑
　e. the information recorded in step 1　❑

EXAMPLE

"This is Sandy Smith, health unit coordinator, orthopedic floor, 3 East at College Hospital. Mary Copa's nurse, Judy Jones, has asked me to inform Dr. Hurtte that Mary Copa's temperature is 38.2 degrees centigrade."

8. Record the time of call and the name of the person you spoke to on the note pad. ❑

9. Notify Judy Jones, RN, that you have placed the call. ❑

Place a check mark (✔) in the box below to indicate that you have completed Activity 4–4.

❑ Place a Telephone Call to a Doctor's Office   Date: _____

ACTIVITY 4-5
LEAVE A VOICE MAIL MESSAGE

Materials Needed   Telephone
Recorder

Situation

The nurse manager, Pat Harris, has requested that you call and leave a voice mail message on Keith Jackson's telephone recorder. The message is that he is cancelled for the night shift tonight and that he is to call her in the morning.

Directions

Practice leaving a voice mail message on a recorder using the information above. Follow the steps below. Place a check mark (✔) in the box as you complete each step.

Steps for Leaving a Voice Mail Message

1. Dial the telephone number supplied to you by your instructor. ❑

2. After listening to the recorded greeting and indicated tone, record your name, hospital name, the nursing unit, the time, and the message, speaking slowly and distinctly. ❑

3. State the nurse manager's name and telephone number during the message and repeat the name and number at the end of the message. ❑

Place a check mark (✔) in the box below to indicate that you have completed Activity 4–5.

❑ Leave a Voice Mail Message   Date: _____

ACTIVITY 4-6
CONTACT A PERSON USING A DIGITAL PAGER

Materials Needed   Digital pager
Telephone
List of pager numbers

Situation

Mary Smith, RN, asks you to page the hospitalist regarding the blood sugar results of Sam Aritan.

Directions

Practice contacting a person using a digital pager using the information in the previous situation. Follow the steps below. Place a check mark (✓) in the box as you complete each step.

Steps for Contacting a Person Using a Digital Pager

1. Record the following information on the note pad: ❑

NOTE PAD

Person to be paged: _____

Pager number: _____

Your telephone number: _____

Time of page: _____

_____

Note: It may be necessary to obtain an outside line when paging a person outside the hospital before proceeding with the remaining steps.

2. Dial the pager number from a touch-tone telephone. ❑

3. Listen for a ring followed by a series of beeps. ❑

4. Dial your telephone number followed by a pound sign (#) to display your number on the pager. Some hospitals use a code number indicating urgency for return call (1 = stat, 2 = ASAP) that is entered after the return number. ❑

5. Listen for a series of beeps or a voice "thank you" message, which indicates a completed page. ❑

Place a check mark (✔) in the box below to indicate that you have completed Activity 4–6.

❑ Contact a Person Using a Digital Pager   Date: _____

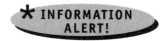

★ INFORMATION ALERT!

In some health care facilities on certain units nurses may carry cellular phones. Calls may be transferred to the nurse's phone, or he or she may receive calls directly from the doctor's office.

Personal and Professional Skills

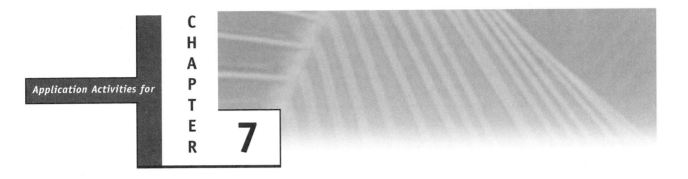

Management Techniques and Problem-Solving Skills for Health Unit Coordinating

Activity in This Chapter

7-1: Prepare a Unit Census Worksheet

ACTIVITY 7-1

PREPARE A UNIT CENSUS WORKSHEET

Materials Needed   Pen or pencil

Unit census worksheet or

Computer and Practice Activity Software for Transcription of Physicians' Orders

Situation

You are the health unit coordinator for the morning shift on a surgical unit at County General Hospital. Nancy Clary, RN, has left the following tape-recorded change-of-shift report as her night shift ended.

Note: A health unit coordinator may listen to the nurse's report or may receive a report from the health unit coordinator going off duty.

Change-of-Shift Report

Joseph Smith (room 401, bed 1) is a 42-year-old with a diagnosis of diabetes mellitus, admitted with gangrene of right foot. He is scheduled for an amputation of right leg up to the knee tomorrow morning. Joe had a good night, but is quite depressed. His blood sugar has been in normal range and he has had his 6:00 AM insulin this morning. Dr. Franks has requested that Joe's AM labs be called to his office today.

Peter Jones (room 401, bed 2) is a 20-year-old admitted with appendicitis at 3:00 AM this morning. He has signed his surgery consent and will be going to surgery to follow the 7:30 AM case. There is a pre-op ordered on call. He has slept off and on since admission, and his girlfriend will be back prior to his surgery. He seems to be a little apprehensive about going to surgery. This is his first hospital admission.

Sally Forest (room 402, bed 1) is a 28-year-old who was admitted 2 days ago after a motor vehicle accident. She had a concussion, fractured ribs, and minor cuts and bruises. Dr. Jones has written her discharge for this morning.

Tillie Frankel (room 402, bed 2) is a 70-year-old admitted last Thursday, diagnosis of cerebral vascular accident. Tillie is still on O_2 at 2 L/min per nasal prongs, has an IV of lactated Ringer's running, and has had a pretty quiet night. She had urinary incontinence twice during the night. She is afebrile. Her total intake during the night was 1450 cc and output approximately 800 cc. Physical therapy will be doing passive exercises this morning. Her husband stayed in her room last night and has requested that no other visitors be allowed.

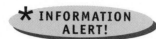

✱ INFORMATION ALERT!

Each nurse will give a report (in person or tape recorded) on the patients that he or she was in charge of during the previous shift. Information will include patient name, room and bed number, age, diagnosis, reason for admission, date and type of surgery if applicable, significant changes during the last 24 hours, tests and procedures during the last shift, tests and procedures for the upcoming shift, important laboratory data, current physical and emotional assessments, vital signs if abnormal, intake and output, IV fluid status, activity, discharge planning, and an update on changes or effectiveness of care plan. The HUC will write down only the information that would be necessary to track patients and their activities and aid in performing required duties and tasks related to the patients.

Directions

Practice preparing a unit census worksheet using the information in the above situation. Follow the steps below. Place a check mark (✓) in the box as you complete each step.

Steps for Preparing a Unit Census Sheet

1. Print a unit census worksheet from the Practice Activity Software for Transcription of Physicians' Orders by choosing *census* from the master screen, and then choosing *census worksheet units A and B.* (If not available, use the patient activity sheet from Appendix B in this book. Write out the room numbers and patient names.) ❑

2. Have someone read the change-of-shift report to you while you record pertinent information on the unit census worksheet. ❑

3. Record the following information for each patient next to his or her name:
   a. any scheduled diagnostic procedure or surgery ❑
   b. any planned discharge, transfer, or admission ❑
   c. do-not-resuscitate (DNR) order ❑
   d. no visitors allowed ❑
   e. do not release information ❑
   f. isolation procedures ❑
   g. no telephone calls allowed ❑
   h. special reports that need to be placed on chart ❑
   i. calling information, such as laboratory results, to doctor's office when available ❑

Place a check mark (✔) in the box below to indicate that you have completed Activity 7–1.

❑ Prepare a Unit Census Worksheet　　　　　Date: _____

The Patient's Chart and Transcription of Doctors' Orders

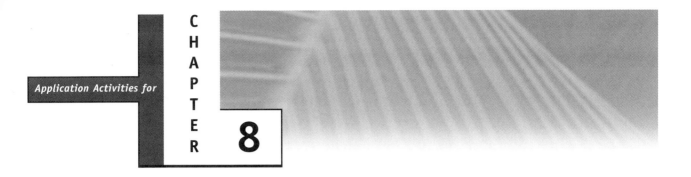

C
H
A
P
T
E
R

Application Activities for

8

The Patient's Chart

Activities in this Chapter

8–1: Convert Standard Time to Military Time and Military Time to Standard Time
8–2: Prepare a Patient's Chart
8–3: Prepare a Consent Form
8–4: Correct an Imprinter/Labeling Error on a Chart Form
8–5: Correct a Written Error on a Chart Form

ACTIVITY 8-1

CONVERT STANDARD TIME TO MILITARY TIME AND MILITARY TIME TO STANDARD TIME

Materials Needed   Pen or pencil

Directions

Convert the listed standard times in the first column to military times. Convert the listed military times in the second column to standard times. Refer to the clock illustration on page 16 as needed. Follow all steps. Place a check mark (✓) in the box as you complete each step.

Column 1		Column 2	
1. 12:00 (noon)	_____	1. 2400	_____
2. 1:15 PM	_____	2. 2119	_____
3. 6:27 AM	_____	3. 0001	_____
4. 4:13 PM	_____	4. 0820	_____
5. 7:05 AM	_____	5. 1919	_____
6. 1:35 AM	_____	6. 0605	_____
7. 11:30 PM	_____	7. 2000	_____
8. 2:00 PM	_____	8. 0900	_____
9. 8:25 PM	_____	9. 1200	_____
10. 5:15 PM	_____	10. 1700	_____

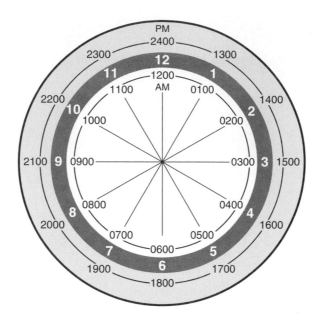

Steps for Converting Standard Time to Military Time and Military Time to Standard Time

1. Enter corresponding military time on the line next to the standard time in column 1:

   a. written with four spaces (example: 9:00 = 0900; 12:00 noon = 1200)

   b. spaces one and two designate the hour and spaces three and four designate the minutes
      (AM and PM are not used)

   c. hours after midnight are 0100 to 1200

   d. a zero is used before the hours 1:00 through 9:00 to provide four spaces (0100 through 0900)

   e. twelve noon is written as 1200 and the hours that follow are arrived at by adding that number
      to 1200 (example: 1200 + 6 as in 6 PM = 1800)

2. Enter corresponding standard time on the line next to military time in column 2:

   a. written with colon and AM to designate hours between 12 midnight and 12 noon
      or PM to designate hours between 12 noon and 12 midnight

   b. hours between 12 midnight and 12 noon may be recognized by the "0" in the first space

   c. hours that follow 12 noon may be arrived at by subtracting 1200 (example:
      1400 − 1200 = 200 = 2:00 PM)

   d. twelve midnight is considered 12:00 AM and twelve noon is considered 12:00 PM

Place a check mark (✔) in the box below to indicate that you have completed Activity 8–1.

☐ Convert Standard Time to Military Time and Military   Date: _____
    Time to Standard Time

✱ INFORMATION ALERT!

The use of military time eliminates confusion because hours are not repeated and the use of AM and PM is unnecessary.

ACTIVITY 8-2

PREPARE A PATIENT'S CHART

Materials Needed   Pens
Patient ID labels
Chart binder and dividers
Patient chart forms listed in step 1
Computer and Practice Activity Software for Transcription of Physicians' Orders

Directions

Prepare a patient's chart by following the steps below. Check with your instructor for variations of the procedure to adapt it to the practice in your area. Place a check mark (✓) in the box as you complete each step.

Steps for Preparing a Patient's Chart

1. Remove the following standard patient chart forms from Appendix B, or print out the forms from the CD-ROM practice software.
   a. Condition of Agreement form (COA or C of A)—(initiated in the admitting department) ☐
   b. Information Sheet (Face Sheet)—(initiated in the admitting department) ☐
   c. Advance Directive Checklist—(initiated in the admitting department) ☐
   d. Physician's Order Form ☐
   e. Physician's Progress Record ☐
   f. Nurse's Admission Record ☐
   g. Nurse's Progress Notes ☐
   h. Graphic Record Form ☐
   i. Medication Administration Record (MAR) ☐
   j. Nurse's Discharge-Planning Form ☐
   k. Physician's Discharge Summary ☐
   l. History and Physical (H&P) Form ☐

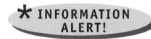 **INFORMATION ALERT!**

Each patient must have a medication administration record (MAR) that an RN will sign off at the end of each shift—even if the patient is not receiving any medication.

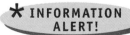 **INFORMATION ALERT!**

For future reference, list any other standard chart forms used in your area.

2. Label each standard chart form with your with patient's ID label. (If labels are not available, write patient information on each form.) You may choose a patient from the list of patients provided in the CD software or create your own patient. To create your own patient, make up a name, an age, and the name of an admitting doctor. ☐

3. Fill in the dates in ink where required on the forms. ☐

4. Label the chart binder with:
   a. the patient's name ☐
   b. the doctor's name ☐
   c. the room and bed numbers ☐

5. Place the completed standard patient chart forms in the patient's chart holder behind the correct divider. ☐

Place a check mark (✔) in the box below to indicate that you have completed Activity 8–2.

☐ Prepare a Patient's Chart   Date: _____

ACTIVITY 8-3

PREPARE A CONSENT FORM

Materials Needed   Patient ID labels
                          Consent form for surgery

Situation

Your patient was admitted to the medical floor at Opportunity Medical Center with a diagnosis of acute appendicitis. Your patient's doctor writes an order for consent for an appendectomy.

Directions

Practice preparing a consent form for surgery using the information in the above situation. Follow the steps below. Check with your instructor for variations of the procedure to adapt it to the practice in your area. Place a check mark (✔) in the box as you complete each step.

Steps for Preparing a Consent Form for Surgery

1. Obtain a surgery consent form for surgery from Appendix B of this book or from the CD-ROM practice software   ☐

2. Label the consent form with the patient's ID label. (If labels are not available, write patient information on consent form.)   ☐

3. Fill in the consent form in ink by writing:
   a. the first and last name of the patient   ☐
   b. the first and last name of the physician   ☐
   c. the surgery or procedure exactly as the doctor wrote it in his or her orders (do not abbreviate)   ☐

✱ **INFORMATION ALERT!**

All written information must be spelled correctly and written legibly. The nurse or physician will fill in the date and time at the time of signing.

4. Place the consent form in the chart binder for reference.   ☐

✱ **INFORMATION ALERT!**

A consent form is also used for medical procedures. Follow the sample steps when filling out a consent form for a medical procedure.

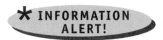

✱ INFORMATION ALERT!

Most health care facilities have a policy that requires a licensed health care provider to witness the signing of a consent form. Telephone consents require two witnesses who will listen to verbal consent given over the telephone. Both will sign as witnesses on the consent form.

Place a check mark (✔) in the box below to indicate that you have completed Activity 8–3.

☐ Prepare a Consent Form   Date: _____

ACTIVITY 8-4

CORRECT AN IMPRINTER/LABELING ERROR ON A CHART FORM

Materials Needed   Patient ID label
Physician's order sheet

Situation

While you are checking your patient's chart, you discover that the doctor's order sheet has been labeled with the wrong patient's label.

Directions

Practice correcting the labeling error on the form below using the information in the above situation. Use the following steps. Check with your instructor for variations of the procedure to adapt it to the practice in your area. Place a check mark (✔) in the box as you complete each step.

963 997 MR 426-743
Breath, Les
Albert Hart
M 40 Surg HMO

PHYSICIANS' ORDER SHEET

Date	Time	Symbol	Orders

Steps for Correcting an Imprinter/Labeling Error on a Chart Form

1. Label with your patient ID label, or write the correct information in ink next to the error. ☐
2. Place an "X" in ink through the incorrect information. ☐
3. Record the words "mistaken entry" in ink above the error. ☐

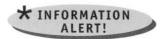

★ INFORMATION ALERT!

Following proper procedure to correct an error on the patient's chart is important, because the chart is a legal document and may be used as evidence in a court of law.

4. Record the date, time, your first initial, your last name, and your status next to the words "mistaken entry."

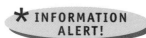

★ INFORMATION ALERT!

Do not place the correct patient ID label over the incorrect label. The correct label could easily be peeled off or fall off the form.

Place a check mark (✔) in the box below to indicate that you have completed Activity 8–4.

☐ Correct a Labeling Error on a Chart Form   Date: _____

ACTIVITY 8-5

CORRECT A WRITTEN ERROR ON A CHART FORM

Materials Needed   Black ink pen

Situation

The physician writes an order for Xanax .25 mg PO q 6 h prn anxiety. You mistakenly write the order on the medication sheet as "Zantac."

Directions

Practice correcting a written error on the chart form below, using the information in the above situation. Follow the steps below. Check with your instructor for variations of the procedure to adapt it to the practice in your area. Place a check mark (✔) in the box as you complete each step.

MEDICATION RECORD							Room No.			Room No.			Room No.		
							Last Name			Last Name			Last Name		
							P.O. Day			P.O. Day			P.O. Day		
	Date	Drug	Dose	Route	Date DC	Schedule	Date *0/0/00*			Date *0/0/00*			Date *0/0/00*		
							11-7	7-3	3-11	11-7	7-3	3-11	11-7	7-3	3-11
1	*0/00*	*Zantac*	*.25mg*	IV (PO) R IM		*prn* *q6h anxiety*									
2				IV PO R IM											
3				IV PO R IM											
4				IV PO R IM											

Steps for Correcting a Written Error on a Chart Form

1. Draw one single line in ink through the error.   ❏

> ✱ **INFORMATION ALERT!**
>
> When only a single line is used to cancel the error, the original recorded information is still readable. When correcting an error on the medication record, the line is drawn through the order date and the name of the medication and to the end of the documentation dates.

2. Record the words "mistaken entry" in ink above or next to the error.   ❏

3. Record the date, time, your first initial, your last name, and your status in a blank area near the words "mistaken entry."   ❏

4. Write the correct order on line 2.   ❏

Place a check mark (✔) in the box below to indicate that you have completed Activity 8–5.

❏ Correct a Written Error on a Chart Form   Date: _____

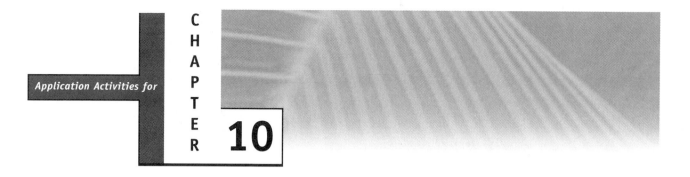

C
H
A
P
T
E
R
10

Patient Activity, Patient Positioning, and Nursing Observation Orders

Place the Physicians' Order Sheets located at the end of the chapter in your patient's chart. Follow the directions for each activity to transcribe orders.

Activities in this Chapter

10–1: Transcribe a Patient Activity Order
10–2: Transcribe a Patient Positioning Order
10–3: Transcribe Nursing Observation Orders
10–4: Automatically Cancel and Discontinue a Doctor's Orders
10–5: Transcribe a Review Set of Doctors' Orders
10–6: Record Telephoned Doctor's Orders
10–7: Record Telephone Messages

 ACTIVITY 10-1

TRANSCRIBE A PATIENT ACTIVITY ORDER

Materials Needed Black ink pen
Red ink pen (depending on hospital policy)
Pencil
Eraser
Kardex form

Directions

Refer to Physicians' Order Sheet 10–1 in your patient's chart. Label or write your patient's name at the top of the order sheet. Write the date and time in the left column next to the first order and sign your patient's doctor's name next to Dr. at the bottom of the order sheet. Practice transcribing the patient activity order by following the steps below. (Check with your instructor for variations of the procedure to adapt the procedure to the practice in your area.) Place a check mark (✓) in the box as you complete each step.

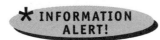

Recite all 10 steps of transcription to yourself as you transcribe the orders to ensure that you do not miss a step. Not every set of orders requires all 10 steps.

Steps for Transcribing a Patient Activity Order

1. Read the order. ☐

2. Obtain the Kardex form. ☐

3. Kardex the order by: ☐
   a. writing the date and the activity order in pencil in the activity column on the Kardex form.
   b. writing the symbol "K" in ink in front of the order on the doctor's order sheet to indicate completion of the kardexing step. ☐

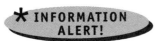

The Kardex form used in this activity will be used through Chapter 18. You will be erasing, changing, and adding information as the doctor's orders are transcribed. It is important to write small, neatly, and legibly and to have a no. 2 pencil with a good eraser or a separate eraser.

4. Recheck each step for accuracy. ☐

5. Sign-off the order in ink by writing the following on the line directly below the doctor's signature: ☐
   a. the date (begin on the left margin) ☐
   b. the time ☐
   c. your full signature ☐
   d. your status ☐

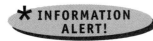

Color of ink used to document completion of transcription steps may be black or red (depends on hospital policy). Blue is not used because it does not copy well on microfilm.

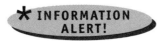

Signing-off the order on the line directly below the doctor's signature avoids leaving space that could be used by the doctor to write additional orders at a later date that could be overlooked.

Place a check mark (✔) in the box below to indicate that you have completed Activity 10–1.

☐ Transcribe a Patient Activity Order   Date: _____

ACTIVITY 10-2

TRANSCRIBE A PATIENT POSITIONING ORDER

Materials Needed   Black ink pen
Red ink pen (depending on hospital policy)
Pencil
Eraser
Kardex form

Directions

Refer to Physicians' Order Sheet 10–2 in your patient's chart. Write the date and time in the left column next to the first order and sign your patient's doctor's name next to Dr. at the bottom of the order sheet. Practice transcribing the patient activity order by following the steps below. (Check with your instructor for variations of the procedure to adapt the procedure to the practice in your area.) Place a check mark (✔) in the box as you complete each step.

Steps for Transcribing a Patient Positioning Order

1. Read the order.   ☐

2. Obtain the Kardex form.   ☐

3. Kardex the order by:
  a. writing the date and the positioning order in pencil in the activity column on the
     Kardex form   ☐
  b. writing the symbol "K" in ink in front of the order on the doctor's order sheet to indicate
     completion of the kardexing step   ☐

4. Recheck each step for accuracy   ☐

5. Sign-off the order in ink by writing the following on the line directly below the doctor's signature
     (begin on the left margin):
  a. the date   ☐
  b. the time   ☐
  c. your full signature   ☐
  d. your status   ☐

Place a check mark (✔) in the box below to indicate that you have completed Activity 10–2.

☐ Transcribe a Patient Positioning Order   Date: _____

ACTIVITY 10-3

TRANSCRIBE NURSING OBSERVATION ORDERS

Materials Needed   Black ink pen

Red ink pen (depending on hospital policy)

Pencil

Eraser

Kardex form

Directions

Refer to Physicians' Order Sheet 10–3 in your patient's chart. Write the date and time in the left column next to the first order and sign your patient's doctor's name next to Dr. at the bottom of the order sheet. Practice transcribing the patient activity order by following the steps below. (Check with your instructor for variations of the procedure to adapt the procedure to the practice in your area.) Place a check mark (✓) in the box as you complete each step.

Steps for Transcribing Nursing Observation Orders

1. Read the orders. ❑

2. Obtain the Kardex form. ❑

3. Kardex the orders by:

a. writing the date and orders in pencil in the appropriate column on the Kardex form (usually the column has the same heading as the doctor's order sheet). ❑

b. writing the symbol "K" in ink in front of the orders on the doctor's order sheet to indicate completion of the kardexing step. ❑

4. Recheck each step for accuracy. ❑

5. Sign-off the orders in ink by writing the following on the line directly below the doctor's signature:

a. the date (begin on the left margin) ❑

b. the time ❑

c. your full signature ❑

d. your status ❑

Place a check mark (✓) in the box below to indicate that you have completed Activity 10–3.

❑ Transcribe Nursing Observation Orders   Date: _____

ACTIVITY 10-4

AUTOMATICALLY CANCEL AND DISCONTINUE DOCTORS' ORDERS

Materials Needed   Black ink pen

Red ink pen (depending on hospital policy)

Pencil

Eraser

Kardex form used in Activity 10–3

Directions

Refer to Physicians' Order Sheet 10–4 in your patient's chart. Write the date and time in the left column next to the first order and sign your patient's doctor's name next to Dr. at the bottom of the order sheet. Practice transcribing the patient activity order by following the steps below. (Check with your instructor for variations of the procedure to adapt the procedure to the practice in your area.) Place a check mark (✓) in the box as you complete each step.

Steps for Automatically Canceling and Discontinuing a Doctor's Orders

1. Read the orders. ❏

2. Obtain the Kardex form. ❏

3. Kardex the discontinued orders by:
   a. erasing the existing date and order. ❏
   b. writing the symbol "K" in ink in front of the order on the doctor's order sheet to indicate completion of the kardexing step ❏

4. Kardex the automatically canceled orders by:
   a. erasing the existing date and order. ❏

✱ INFORMATION ALERT!

When a doctor changes an order, the new order will automatically cancel the existing order.

---

   b. writing the date and new order in pencil in the appropriate column on the Kardex form. ❏
   c. writing the symbol "K" in ink in front of the order on the doctor's order sheet to indicate completion of the kardexing step. ❏

5. Recheck each step for accuracy. ❏

6. Sign-off the orders in ink by writing the following on the line directly below the doctor's signature:
   a. the date (begin at the left margin) ❏
   b. the time ❏
   c. your full signature ❏
   d. your status ❏

Place a check mark (✔) in the box below to indicate that you have completed Activity 10–4.

❏ Automatically Cancel and Discontinue a Doctor's Orders   Date: _____

ACTIVITY 10-5

TRANSCRIBE A REVIEW SET OF DOCTORS' ORDERS

Materials Needed   Black ink pen
                        Red ink pen (depending on hospital policy)
                        Pencil
                        Eraser
                        Kardex form used in Activity 10–4

Directions

Refer to Physicians' Order Sheet 10–5 in your patient's chart. Transcribe the orders. Refer to previous activities for the appropriate directions to prepare for the transcription.

Steps for Transcribing a Review Set of Doctors' Orders

1. Read the orders. ❏

2. Obtain all necessary forms. ❏

> Suggestion to the student: Use this space to list the forms you will need.

3. Kardex the orders. ❏

4. Recheck each step for accuracy. ❏

5. Sign-off the orders to indicate completion of transcription. ❏

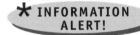 **INFORMATION ALERT!**

Transcribing doctors' orders is a critical task, and an error could cause harm to a patient. If you are not absolutely sure in interpreting a doctor's orders, ask the patient's nurse or the doctor who wrote the orders.

Place a check mark (✔) in the box below to indicate that you have completed Activity 10–5.

❏ Transcribe a Review Set of Doctors' Orders   Date: _____

 ACTIVITY 10-6

RECORD TELEPHONED DOCTORS' ORDERS

Note: Recording telephoned doctors' orders is discussed in Chapter 9 of *Health Unit Coordinating.* Activities providing practice recording telephoned doctors' orders will assist you in learning abbreviations and will be included in this chapter and subsequent chapters through Chapter 18.

Materials Needed

Black ink pen
Physician's order sheet

Directions

Practice recording the telephoned doctor's orders printed below by following the listed steps. Place a check mark (✔) in the box as you complete each step.

Telephoned Doctor's Orders

"Hello, this is Dr. Pete Johnson with orders on a new admit by the name of Mary Copa.
Diagnosis: chronic obstructive pulmonary disease
Complete bed rest with head of bed elevated 30 degrees
Bathroom privileges only
Head of bed elevated thirty degrees when in bed
Vital signs every shift
Blood pressure three times a day standing, sitting, and lying
Record intake and output
Thank you."

Steps for Recording Telephoned Doctor's Orders

1. Have someone read the above orders to you while you record them on a doctor's order form. ❑

2. Use accepted abbreviations and symbols as you write the orders. ❑

3. Follow the guidelines provided in Chapter 9 of *Health Unit Coordinating*. ❑

4. For further practice, obtain a new Kardex form and practice transcribing the orders that you have written. ❑

Place a check mark (✔) in the box below to indicate that you have completed Activity 10–6.

❑ Record Telephoned Doctors' Orders   Date: _____

ACTIVITY 10-7

RECORD TELEPHONE MESSAGES

Note: Recording telephone messages is an important part of the health unit coordinator's job. Activities will be provided for practice in recording messages will be provided in this chapter and in subsequent chapters through Chapter 18.

Materials Needed   Pen or pencil
                          Message pad

Directions

Practice recording the telephone messages printed below by following the steps listed below. Place a check mark (✓) in the box as you complete each step.

Telephone Messages

1. "Hello, this is Dr. Peterson. Would you ask Mrs. Johnson's nurse (Diane) to call me for orders regarding medication changes? My back office number is 345-4980. Thank you." ❑

2. "Hi, this is Jamie from Dr. Sanburn's office. Dr. Sanburn would like the nurse to call regarding Johnny Appleton. Our number is 596-3249." ❑

Steps for Recording Telephone Messages

1. Have someone read the above messages to you while you record them on a message pad. ❑

2. Write down who the message is for. ❑

3. Write down the caller's name. ❑

4. Write down the date and time of the call. ❑

5. Write down the purpose of the call. ❑

6. If a return call is expected, write down the number to call. ❑

7. Sign your name to the message. ❑

Place a check mark (✔) in the box below to indicate that you have completed Activity 10–7.

☐ Record Telephone Messages   Date: _____

PHYSICIANS' ORDER SHEET 10–1

DATE	TIME	SYMBOL	ORDERS
			CBR
			Dr

PHYSICIANS' ORDER SHEET 10–2

DATE	TIME	SYMBOL	ORDERS
			↑ HoB 30°
			TCDB q 2 hr
			Dr

PHYSICIANS' ORDER SHEET 10–3

DATE	TIME	SYMBOL	ORDERS
			Wt daily
			vs q 4 hr until stable
			strict I & O
			Dr

PHYSICIANS' ORDER SHEET 10–4

DATE	TIME	SYMBOL	ORDERS
			D/C q 4° vs
			D/C I & O
			Up in chair x 20 min this pm
			WT qod—may stand @ bedside
			Dr

PHYSICIANS' ORDER SHEET 10–5

DATE	TIME	SYMBOL	ORDERS
			↑ lt arm on 2 pillows x 24°
			CMS lt fingers q 2° x 24°
			NVS q 4° x 12°
			Dr

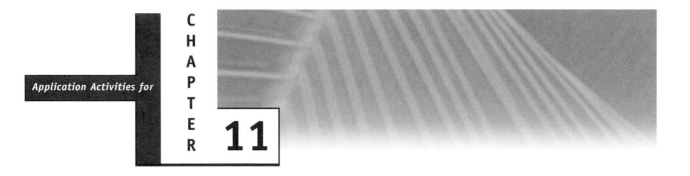

Nursing Treatment Orders

Place the Physicians' Order Sheets located at the end of the chapter in your patient's chart. Follow the directions for each activity to transcribe orders.

Activities in this Chapter

ACTIVITY 11-1

TRANSCRIBE URINARY CATHETERIZATION AND INTESTINAL ELIMINATION ORDERS

Materials Needed: Black ink pen
Red ink pen (depending on hospital policy)
Pencil
Eraser
Kardex form used in Chapter 10

Directions

Refer to Physicians' Order Sheet 11–1 in your patient's chart. Practice transcribing the nursing treatment orders by following the steps below. Check with your instructor for variations of the procedure to adapt it to the practice in your area. Place a check mark (✓) in the box as you complete each step.

Steps for Transcribing Urinary Catheterization and Intestinal Elimination Orders

1. Read the orders.   ❏

2. Obtain the Kardex form used in Chapter 10.   ❏

3. Kardex the orders by:
   a. writing the date and order in pencil in the treatment column on the Kardex form.   ❏
   b. writing the symbol "K" in ink in front of the order on the doctor's order sheet to indicate
      completion of the kardexing step.   ❏

4. Recheck each step for accuracy.   ❏

5. Sign-off the orders to indicate completion of transcription.   ❏

Place a check mark (✔) in the box below to indicate that you have completed Activity 11-1.

❏ Transcribe Urinary Catheterization and Intestinal
  Elimination Orders   Date: _____

ACTIVITY 11-2

TRANSCRIBE INTRAVENOUS THERAPY ORDERS

Materials Needed   Black ink pen

Red ink pen (depending on hospital policy)

Pencil

Eraser

Kardex form used in Activity 11–1

Patient ID labels (if using the requisition method)

Central Service Department (CSD) requisition (if using the requisition method)

Computer and Practice Activity Software for Transcription of Physicians' Orders

Directions

Refer to Physicians' Order Sheet 11–2 in your patient's chart. Practice transcribing the nursing treatment orders by following the steps below. Check with your instructor for variations of the procedure to adapt it to the practice in your area. Place a check mark (✓) in the box as you complete each step.

Steps for Transcribing Intravenous Therapy Orders

1. Read the orders.   ❏

2. Obtain the Kardex form and CSD requisition form if using the requisition method.   ❏

3. Order an IV infusion pump.   ❏

Use the computer method by:
   a. selecting Enter Orders on the master screen   ❏
   b. selecting the patient's name from the census on the viewing screen.   ❏
   c. selecting the CSD from the department menu on the viewing screen.   ❏
   d. selecting the IV infusion pump from the menu on the viewing screen.   ❏
   e. typing in the pertinent information.   ❏
   f. writing "ord" IV pump above the IV order on the doctor's order sheet to indicate
      that the IV equipment has been ordered.   ❏

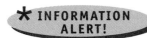

★ INFORMATION ALERT!

When using the computer method in the hospital to complete the ordering step during the transcription process, you would press "enter" after completing the order screen to send the order to the appropriate department. A "hard copy" of the order may also print on the nursing unit printer.

Use the requisition method by:
a. labeling the requisition.
b. filling in the pertinent information.
c. placing the number "1" in the box next to IV infusion pump (in ink).
d. writing "ord IV pump" above the IV order on the doctor's order sheet to indicate that the IV equipment has been ordered.

4. Kardex the orders by:
a. writing the date and the order in pencil in the intravenous (IV) column on the Kardex form.
b. writing the symbol "K" in ink in front of the order on the doctor's order sheet to indicate completion of the kardexing step.

5. Recheck each step for accuracy.

6. Sign-off the orders to indicate completion of transcription.

★ INFORMATION ALERT!

Some hospitals may use a parenteral fluid or infusion form to record IV orders, and some may write the IV orders on the MAR.

Place a check mark (✔) in the box below to indicate that you have completed Activity 11–2.

☐ Transcribe Intravenous Therapy Orders   Date: _____

➤ **ACTIVITY 11-3**

TRANSCRIBE SUCTION ORDERS

Materials Needed   Black ink pen

Red ink pen (depending on hospital policy)

Pencil

Eraser

Kardex form used in Activity 11–2

Patient ID label (if using the requisition method)

CSD requisition (if using the requisition method)

List of items that may be stored in the CSD (See Table 11–1 in *Health Unit Coordinating*, 5th edition)

Computer and Practice Activity Software for Transcription of Physicians' Orders

Directions

Refer to Physicians' Order Sheet 11–3 in your patient's chart. Practice transcribing the nursing treatment orders by following the steps below. Check with your instructor for variations of the procedure to adapt it to the practice in your area. Place a check mark (✓) in the box as you complete each step.

Steps for Transcribing Suction Orders

1. Read the orders. ❏

2. Obtain the Kardex form and CSD requisition form if using the requisition method. ❏

> **✳ INFORMATION ALERT!**
>
> Refer to Table 11–1 in *Health Unit Coordinating,* 5th edition, to determine the supplies and equipment that may need to be ordered.

3. Order the supplies and equipment from the CSD. ❏

Use the computer method by:
a. selecting Enter Orders from the master screen ❏
b. selecting the patient's name from the census on the viewing screen. ❏
c. selecting the CSD from the department menu on the viewing screen. ❏
d. selecting the item(s) to be ordered from the menu on the viewing screen and typing in the pertinent information. ❏
e. sending the order by pressing "enter" on the computer keyboard. ❏
f. writing "ord" above each order on the doctor's order sheet to indicate that all equipment has been ordered. ❏

Use the requisition method by:
a. labeling the requisition with the patient's label. ❏
b. filling in the pertinent information. ❏
c. placing an "X" or a quantity (if applicable) in the column next to the item(s) to be ordered. ❏
d. writing "ord" in ink above any item ordered on the doctor's order sheet to indicate that the item was ordered. ❏

4. Kardex the orders by:
a. writing the date and order in pencil in the treatment column on the Kardex form. ❏
b. writing the symbol "K" in ink in front of the order on the doctor's order sheet to indicate completion of the kardexing step. ❏

5. Recheck each step for accuracy. ❏

6. Sign-off the orders to indicate completion of transcription. ❏

Place a check mark (✓) in the box below to indicate that you have completed Activity 11–3.

❏ Transcribe Suction Orders   Date: _____

ACTIVITY 11-4

TRANSCRIBE HEAT AND COLD APPLICATION ORDERS AND COMFORT, SAFETY, AND HEALING ORDERS

Materials Needed   Black ink pen
Red ink pen (depending on hospital policy)
Pencil
Eraser
Kardex form used in Activity 11–3

Patient ID labels (when using the requisition method)

CSD requisition (when using the requisition method)

Computer and Practice Activity Software for Transcription of Physicians' Orders

Directions

Refer to Physicians' Order Sheet 11–4 in your patient's chart. Practice transcribing the nursing treatment orders by following the steps below. Check with your instructor for variations of the procedure to adapt it to the practice in your area. Place a check mark (✓) in the box as you complete each step.

Steps for Transcribing Heat and Cold Application Orders and Comfort, Safety, and Healing Orders

1. Read the orders. ❑

2. Obtain the Kardex form and CSD requisition form if using the requisition method. ❑

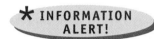

> Refer to Table 11–1 in *Health Unit Coordinating*, 5th edition, to determine the supplies and equipment that may need to be ordered.

3. Order the supplies and equipment from the CSD. ❑

Use the computer method by:
a. selecting Enter Orders from the master screen ❑
b. selecting the patient's name from the census on the viewing screen. ❑
c. selecting the CSD from the department menu on the viewing screen. ❑
d. selecting the item(s) to be ordered from the menu on the viewing screen. ❑
e. typing in the pertinent information. ❑
f. sending the order by pressing "enter" on the computer keyboard. ❑
g. writing "ord" in ink above each order on the doctor's
order sheet to indicate that supplies and equipment have been ordered. ❑

Use the requisition method by:
a. labeling with patient ID label. ❑
b. filling in the pertinent information. ❑
c. placing an "X" or a quantity (if applicable) in the column next to the item(s) to be ordered. ❑
d. writing "ord" in ink above each order on the doctor's order sheet to indicate that supplies
and equipment have been ordered. ❑

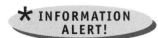

> Writing "ord" above each item ordered will reduce the risk of missing items. When the computer method is being used, the computer order number is often written above items to indicate that they have been ordered.
> Example: ord
> K-pad to lower lt arm 20 min qid

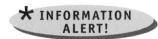

> Check with your instructor for the size of the Ted hose (Teds) to be ordered.

4. Kardex the orders by:
   a. writing the date and order in pencil in the treatment column on the Kardex form. ❑
   b. writing the symbol "K" in ink in front of the order on the doctor's order sheet to indicate completion of the kardexing step. ❑
5. Recheck each step for accuracy. ❑
6. Sign-off the orders to indicate completion of transcription. ❑

Place a check mark (✓) in the box below to indicate that you have completed Activity 11–4.

❑ Transcribe Heat and Cold Application Orders
and Comfort, Safety, and Healing Orders   Date: _____

ACTIVITY 11-5

TRANSCRIBE A BLOOD GLUCOSE MONITORING ORDER

Materials Needed   Black ink pen
                        Red ink pen (depending on hospital policy)
                        Pencil
                        Eraser
                        Kardex form used in Activity 11–4

Directions

Refer to Physicians' Order Sheet 11–5 in your patient's chart. Practice transcribing the nursing treatment order by following the steps below. Check with your instructor for variations of the procedure to adapt it to the practice in your area. Place a check mark (✓) in the box as you complete each step.

Steps for Transcribing a Blood Glucose Monitoring Order

1. Read the order. ❑
2. Obtain the Kardex form. ❑
3. Kardex the order by:
   a. writing the date and the order in pencil in the treatment column on the Kardex form. ❑
   b. writing the symbol "K" in ink in front of the order on the doctor's sheet to indicate completion of the kardexing step. ❑
4. Recheck each step for accuracy. ❑
5. Sign-off the order to indicate completion of transcription. ❑

Place a check mark (✓) in the box below to indicate that you have completed Activity 11–5.

❑ Transcribe a Blood Glucose Monitoring Order   Date: _____

ACTIVITY 11-6

TRANSCRIBE A REVIEW SET OF DOCTORS' ORDERS

Materials Needed　　Black ink pen

Red ink pen (depending on hospital policy)

Pencil

Eraser

Kardex form used in Activity 11–5

Patient ID label (if using requisition method)

Necessary requisitions (if using requisition method)

Computer and Practice Activity Software for Transcription of Physicians' Orders

Directions

Refer to Physicians' Order Sheet 11–6 in your patient's chart. Transcribe the orders. Review the previous activities for the appropriate transcription steps if necessary.

Steps for Transcribing a Review Set of Doctors' Orders

1. Read the orders.　　　　❑

2. Obtain all necessary forms.　　　　❑

> Suggestion to the student: Use this space to list the forms you will need.

3. Order as necessary.　　　　❑

4. Kardex the orders.　　　　❑

5. Recheck each step for accuracy.　　　　❑

6. Sign off the orders to indicate the completion of transcription.　　　　❑

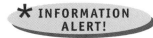

★ INFORMATION ALERT!

Transcribing doctors' orders is a critical task, and an error could cause harm to a patient. If you are not absolutely sure in interpreting the doctor's orders, ask the patient's nurse or the doctor who wrote the orders.

Place a check mark (✓) in the box below to indicate that you have completed Activity 11–6.

☐ Transcribe a Review Set of Doctors' Orders   Date: _____

✱ INFORMATION ALERT!

Refer to *Health Unit Coordinating*, 5th edition (Chapter 11) to determine how long the two bags of IV solution ordered in Activity 11–6 would take to infuse.

ACTIVITY 11-7

RECORD TELEPHONED DOCTORS' ORDERS

Materials Needed   Ink pen
                              Physicians' order sheet

Directions

Practice recording the telephoned doctor's orders printed below by following the steps below. Place a check mark (✓) in the box as you complete each step.

Telephoned Doctors' Orders

"This is Dr. Frank Norstrum with orders on Sally Pike. Ready?
Insert Foley cath
Intermittent CBI every 4 hours times six
Intake and output
Discontinue continuous intravenous fluids and convert to Heplock for intravenous piggyback
    medications
Bathroom privileges with elevated toilet seat
Oil-retention enema in AM
Thank you."

Steps for Recording Telephoned Doctors' Orders

1. Have someone read the above orders to you while you record them on a physicians' order sheet.   ☐

2. Use accepted abbreviations and symbols as you write the orders.   ☐

3. Follow the guidelines provided in Chapter 9 of *Health Unit Coordinating*, 5th Edition.   ☐

4. For further practice, obtain a new Kardex and practice transcribing the orders you have written.   ☐

Place a check mark (✓) in the box below to indicate that you have completed Activity 11–7.

☐ Record Telephoned Doctors' Orders   Date: _____

ACTIVITY 11-8

RECORD TELEPHONE MESSAGES

Materials Needed   Pen or pencil
Message pad

Directions

Practice recording the telephone messages printed below by following the steps below. Place a check mark (✓) in the box as you complete each step.

Telephone Messages

1. "Hello, this is Don in the central service department. Would you ask Mary Copa's nurse for a size on those Ted Hose that were ordered? All the requisition indicated was that they were to be thigh high and we need to know a size." ❑

2. "This is Melba in the pharmacy. Please notify the resident for Peter Franks that we need a clarification on the chemotherapy orders before noon today. Fax them to us as soon as you have them. Thanks." ❑

Steps for Recording Telephone Messages

1. Have someone read the above messages to you while you record them on a message pad. ❑
2. Write down who the message is for. ❑
3. Write down the caller's name. ❑
4. Write down the date and time of the call. ❑
5. Write down the purpose of the call. ❑
6. If a return call is expected, write down the number to call. ❑
7. Sign your name to the message. ❑

Place a check mark (✓) in the box below to indicate that you have completed Activity 11–8.

❑ Record Telephone Messages   Date: _____

PHYSICIANS' ORDER SHEET 11–1

DATE	TIME	SYMBOL	ORDERS
			May have TWE x 1 for gas pains
			Cath q 3° prn if unable to void x 48°
			Fleets enema in am
			Dr

PHYSICIANS' ORDER SHEET 11–2

DATE	TIME	SYMBOL	ORDERS
			Alternate 1000 cc D5W c̄ 1000 cc LR 125 cc/hr
			D/C IV when pt taking po fluids
			Dr

PHYSICIANS' ORDER SHEET 11–3

DATE	TIME	SYMBOL	ORDERS
			Have consent signed for insertion of chest tube rt. side
			Chest tube to Pleur-evac @ 20 cm H_2O suction
			Throat suction @ bedside x 48 hr
			Keep hemovac compressed
			Dr

PHYSICIANS' ORDER SHEET 11–4

DATE	TIME	SYMBOL	ORDERS
			K-pad to lower lt arm 20 min qid
			Ice bag to rt. wrist x 12°
			Alternating pressure pad & footboard
			B/L thigh high Teds
			Dr

PHYSICIANS' ORDER SHEET 11–5

DATE	TIME	SYMBOL	ORDERS
			Accu √AC & HS
			Dr

PHYSICIANS' ORDER SHEET 11–6

DATE	TIME	SYMBOL	ORDERS
			D/C IV's
			D/C footboard
			Up in chair BID c̄ abd elastic binder
			Wt qd @ 0700
			Routine VS
			D/C Teds—pneumatic hose when in bed
			Dr

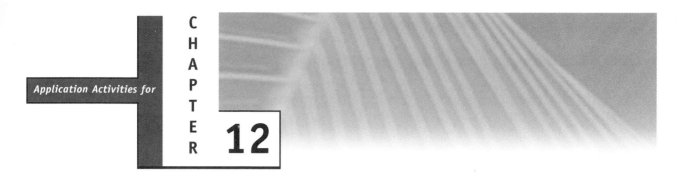

Dietary Orders

Place the Physicians' Order Sheets located at the end of the chapter in your patient's chart. Follow the directions for each activity to transcribe orders.

Activities in this Chapter

 ACTIVITY 12-1

TRANSCRIBE A STANDARD HOSPITAL DIET ORDER

Materials Needed   Black ink pen
Red ink pen (depending on hospital policy)
Pencil
Eraser
Kardex form used in previous chapters
Patient ID label (if requisition method is used)
Diet requisition form (if requisition method is used)
Computer and Practice Activity Software for Transcription of Physicians' Orders

DISCARD

Directions

Refer to Physicians' Order Sheet 12–1 in your patient's chart. Practice transcribing the standard hospital diet by following the steps below. Check with your instructor for variations of the procedure to adapt it to the practice in your area. Place a check mark (✓) in the box as you complete each step.

Steps for Transcribing a Standard Hospital Diet Order

1. Read the order. ❑

2. Obtain the Kardex form used in Chapter 11 and dietary requisition if using the requisition method. ❑

3. Order the diet from the dietary department. ❑

Use the computer method by:
a. selecting Enter Orders on the master screen ❑
b. selecting the patient's name from the census on the viewing screen ❑
c. selecting the dietary department from the department menu on the viewing screen ❑
d. selecting the diet to be ordered from the menu on the viewing screen ❑
e. Typing in the pertinent information ❑
f. sending the order by pressing "enter" on the computer keyboard
g. writing "ord" in ink above the order on the doctor's order sheet to indicate that the diet has been ordered ❑

Use the requisition method by:
a. labeling the dietary requisition with patient ID label ❑
b. writing in the pertinent information ❑
c. placing a check mark (✓) in the column next to the diet to be ordered ❑
d. writing "ord" in ink above the order on the doctor's order sheet to indicate that the diet has been ordered ❑

4. Kardex the order by:
a. writing the date and the order in pencil in the diet column on the Kardex form ❑
b. writing the symbol "K" in ink in front of the order on the doctor's order sheet to indicate completion of the kardexing step ❑

5. Recheck each step for accuracy. ❑

6. Sign-off the order to indicate completion of transcription. ❑

Place a check mark (✓) in the box below to indicate that you have completed Activity 12–1.

❑ Transcribe a Standard Hospital Diet Order Date: _____

ACTIVITY 12-2

TRANSCRIBE A THERAPEUTIC DIET ORDER

Materials Needed Black ink pen

Red ink pen (depending on hospital policy)

Pencil

Eraser

Kardex form used in Activity 12–1

Patient ID label (if requisition method is used)

Diet requisition form (if requisition method is used)

Computer and Practice Activity Software for Transcription of Physicians' Orders

Directions

Refer to Physicians' Order Sheet 12–2 in your patient's chart. Practice transcribing the therapeutic diet order by following the steps below. Check with your instructor for variations of the procedure to adapt it to the practice in your area. Place a check mark (✓) in the box as you complete each step.

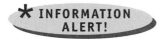

★ INFORMATION ALERT!

An order modifying a nutrient or number of calories would not change the consistency of a patient's diet. Example: If the patient is on a "soft diet" and the doctor wrote an order for "2 g Na," the patient's diet would then be a "soft 2 g Na."

Steps for Transcribing a Therapeutic Diet Order

1. Read the order. ❑

2. Obtain the Kardex form and dietary requisition if using the requisition method. ❑

3. Order the diet from the dietary department. ❑

Use the computer method by:
a. selecting Enter Orders on the master screen ❑
b. selecting the patient's name from the census on the viewing screen ❑
c. selecting the dietary department from the department menu on the viewing screen ❑
d. selecting the diet to be ordered from the menu on the viewing screen ❑
e. typing in the pertinent information ❑
f. sending the order by pressing "enter" on the computer keyboard ❑
g. writing "ord" in ink above the order on the doctor's order sheet to indicate that the diet has been ordered ❑

Use the requisition method by:
a. labeling the dietary requisition with patient's ID label ❑
b. writing in the pertinent information ❑
c. placing a check mark (✓) in the column next to the diet to be ordered ❑
d. writing "ord" in ink above the order on the doctor's order sheet to indicate the diet has been ordered ❑

4. Kardex the order by:
a. writing the date and the order in pencil in the diet column on the Kardex form ❑
b. writing the symbol "K" in ink in front of the order on the doctor's order sheet to indicate completion of the kardexing step ❑

5. Recheck each step for accuracy. ❑

6. Sign-off the order to indicate completion of transcription. ❑

Place a check mark (✔) in the box below to indicate that you have completed Activity 12–2.

❑ Transcribe a Therapeutic Diet Order   Date: _____

ACTIVITY 12-3

TRANSCRIBE A TUBE-FEEDING ORDER

Materials Needed
Black ink pen
Red ink pen (depending on hospital policy)
Pencil
Eraser
Kardex form used in Activity 12–2
Patient's ID label (if using requisition method)
Necessary requisition forms (if using requisition method)
Computer and Practice Activity Software for Transcription of Physicians' Orders

Directions

Refer to Physicians' Order Sheet 12–3 in your patient's chart. Practice transcribing the tube-feeding order by following the steps below. Check with your instructor for variations of the procedure to adapt it to the practice in your area. Place a check mark (✓) in the box as you complete each step.

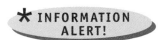

★ **INFORMATION ALERT!**

The nurse may verify the tube placement by withdrawing a small amount of stomach contents or by using a syringe to inject air throught the tube and listening with a stethoscope as the air enters the stomach.

Steps for Transcribing a Feeding-Tube Order

1. Read the order. ❑

2. Obtain the Kardex form and dietary requisition if using the requisition method. ❑

3. Order the feeding pump with bag and tubing from CSD. ❑

4. Order tube-feeding formula from the dietary department. ❑

Use the computer method by:
a. selecting Enter Orders from the master screen ❑
b. selecting the patient's name from the census on the viewing screen ❑
c. selecting the central service department from the department menu on the viewing screen ❑
d. selecting feeding pump with bag and tubing to be ordered
e. typing in the pertinent information
f. sending the order by pressing "enter" on the computer keyboard ❑
g. writing "ord" in ink above the order on the doctor's order sheet to indicate that the feeding pump has been ordered. ❑
h. selecting the dietary department from the department menu on the viewing screen ❑
i. selecting the "Other" option from the menu on the viewing screen and typing out directions for the tube-feeding formula ❑
j. sending the order by pressing "enter" on the computer keyboard ❑
k. writing "ord" in ink above the order on the doctor's order sheet to indicate that the tube-feeding formula has been ordered ❑

Use the requisition method by:
a. labeling the CSD requisition with the patient ID label ❑
b. writing in the pertinent information ❑
c. writing "ord" in ink above the order on the doctor's order sheet to indicate that the feeding pump and tubing have been ordered ❑

d. labeling the dietary requisition with the patient ID label ❑

e. writing in the pertinent information ❑

f. writing "ord" in ink above the order on the doctor's order sheet to indicate
that the tube-feeding formula has been ordered ❑

5. Kardex the order by:

a. writing the date and the order in pencil in the tube-feeding column on the Kardex form ❑

b. writing "K" in ink in front of the order on the doctor's order sheet to indicate completion
of the kardexing step ❑

6. Recheck each step for accuracy. ❑

7. Sign off on the order to indicate completion of transcription. ❑

Place a check mark (✔) in the box below to indicate that you have completed Activity 12–3.

❑ Transcribe a Tube-Feeding Order   Date: _____

ACTIVITY 12-4

TRANSCRIBE A REVIEW SET OF DOCTORS' ORDERS

Materials Needed   Black ink pen

Red ink pen (depending on hospital policy)

Pencil

Eraser

Kardex form used in Activity 12–3

Patient's ID labels (if requisition method is used)

Necessary requisition forms (if requisition method is used)

Necessary consent forms

Directions

Refer to Physicians' Order Sheet 12–4 in your patient's chart. Transcribe the orders. Refer to previous activities for the appropriate transcription steps if necessary.

Steps for Transcribing a Review Set of Doctors' Orders

1. Read the complete set of doctors' orders. ❑

2. Obtain all necessary forms. ❑

Suggestion to the student: Use this space to list the forms you will need.

3. Order as necessary. ☐

4. Kardex the orders. ☐

5. Recheck each step for accuracy. ☐

6. Sign-off the orders to indicate completion of transcription. ☐

✷ INFORMATION ALERT!

Transcribing doctors' orders is a critical task, and an error could cause harm to a patient. If you are not absolutely sure in interpreting the doctor's orders, ask the patient's nurse or the doctor who wrote the orders.

Place a check mark (✔) in the box below to indicate that you have completed Activity 12–4.

☐ Transcribe a Review Set of Doctors' Orders   Date: _____

ACTIVITY 12-5

RECORD TELEPHONED DOCTORS' ORDERS

Materials Needed   Black ink pen
Physicians' order sheet

Directions

Practice recording the telephoned doctors' orders printed below by following the steps below. Place a check mark (✔) in the box as you complete each step.

Telephoned Doctors' Orders

"Hello, this is Dr. Sam Brown with orders on Mary Copa.

Bathroom privileges with bedside commode

Start intravenous fluids of 1000 CCs of 5% dextrose in lactated Ringer's to run at 120 CCs per hour

Diet as tolerated—no added salt

Have dietitian see patient

Soap suds enema tonight, repeat at 0600

Thank you."

Steps for Transcribing Doctors' Orders

1. Have someone read the above orders to you while you record them on a physician's order sheet. ☐

2. Use accepted abbreviations and symbols as you write the orders. ☐

3. Follow the guidelines you have written in Activity 9–1. ☐

4. For further practice, obtain a new Kardex form and practice transcribing the orders you have written. ☐

Place a check mark (✔) in the box below to indicate that you have completed Activity 12–5.

☐ Record Telephoned Doctors' Orders   Date: _____

ACTIVITY 12-6

RECORD TELEPHONE MESSAGES

Materials Needed   Pen or pencil
Message pad

Directions

Practice recording the telephone messages printed below by following the steps below. Place a check mark (✓) in the box as you complete each step.

Telephone Messages

1. "Hello, this is Charlotte Jones, from Adult Protective Services. I'm arranging to have Paula Praline admitted to an adult crisis center. Would you have the case manager call me at 495-3947 as soon as possible? I need to know if Paula is still on a tube feeding or if she has any other dietary restrictions. Thanks."

2. "Hello, this is Dr. Johnson. Would you please advise Mary Copa's nurse that I will be in to do the lumbar puncture at 0830 tomorrow? Please tell her to have Mary Copa sign a consent, and to have the tray with size 8 gloves at the bedside. Thank you."

Steps for Recording Telephone Messages

1. Have someone read the above messages to you while you record them on a message pad. ❑

2. Write down the person's name for whom the message is intended. ❑

3. Write down the caller's name. ❑

4. Write down the date and time of the call. ❑

5. Write down the purpose of the call. ❑

6. If a return call is expected, write down the number to call. ❑

7. Sign your name to the message. ❑

Place a check mark (✔) in the box below to indicate that you have completed Activity 12–6.

❑ Record Telephone Messages   Date: _____

PHYSICIANS' ORDER SHEET 12–1

DATE	TIME	SYMBOL	ORDERS
			soft diet
			Dr

PHYSICIANS' ORDER SHEET 12–2

DATE	TIME	SYMBOL	ORDERS
			2.5 gm Na diet
			Cal ct
			RD consult
			Dr

PHYSICIANS' ORDER SHEET 12–3

DATE	TIME	SYMBOL	ORDERS
			Insert NG feeding tube, verify placement & begin feeding
			of Boost plus initial FS @ 35 cc/hr progress by 10 cc/hr
			q 4 hr as tolerated to final rate of 75 cc/hr
			Dr

PHYSICIANS' ORDER SHEET 12–4

DATE	TIME	SYMBOL	ORDERS
			D/C hemovac c̄ next dressing △
			D/C chest tube
			Amb c̄ help
			BP lying, sitting & standing
			TWE hs
			Cath for residual
			Remove feeding tube & start on cl liq diet, advance DAT
			D/C K-pad
			Insert PICC & start IVF of 0.45 NS @ 120 cc/hr
			Dr
			△ PICC dressing q 8° & report observations
			Dr

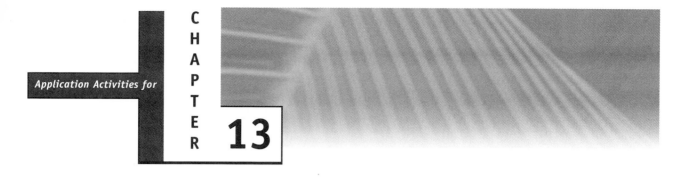

Application Activities for

CHAPTER 13

Medication Orders

Place the Physicians' Order Sheets located at the end of the chapter in your patient's chart. Follow the directions for each activity to transcribe orders.

Activities in this Chapter

ACTIVITY 13-1

TRANSCRIBE STANDING MEDICATION ORDERS

Materials Needed

Black ink pen

Red ink pen (depending on hospital policy)

Pharmacy copy of doctor's orders

PDR or pharmacology reference

Medication time schedule (Table 13–1) in *Health Unit Coordinating*, 5th ed.

Labeled medication administration record (MAR)

Computer and Practice Activity Software for Transcription of Physicians' Orders

Directions

Refer to Physicians' Order Sheet 13–1 in your patient's chart. Practice transcribing the standing medication orders by following the steps below. Check with your instructor for variations of this procedure to adapt it to the practice in your area. Place a check mark (✓) in the box as you complete each step.

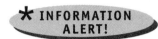

The medication administration record (MAR) used in this activity will be used in all of the following activities. Medications that are not changed or discontinued will be recopied on a new MAR when the dates run out on the current one.

Steps for Transcribing Standing Medication Orders

1. Read the orders.

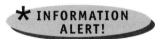

Use the PDR or a pharmacology reference to familiarize yourself with the purpose and correct spelling of the medication.

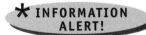

Some medications are administered by one route only. Therefore, the doctor may not include the route of administration when writing the order.

2. Obtain the medication administration record (MAR).

3. Order medications by faxing or sending the pharmacy copy of the doctor's orders to the pharmacy.

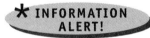

- Medications are ordered by faxing or sending a copy of the doctor's orders to the pharmacy.
- It may not be possible to practice this step in the classroom.
- Follow the next step of writing "faxed pc" or "pcs" with the time and your initials to indicate that you have completed that task.

4. Write "faxed" or "pcs" (pharmacy copy sent) with time and your initials in ink on the doctor's order sheet to indicate that the pharmacy copy has been sent. ❏

✱ INFORMATION ALERT!

It is important to send pharmacy copies or fax doctors' orders to the pharmacy as soon as possible. Medications can then be sent to the floor and be administered to patients. If several charts are flagged, read all orders, transcribe "stat" orders, and send pharmacy copies or fax orders before beginning transcription of orders.

---

5. Enter medications on your patient's medication profile using a computer and the Practice Activity Software for Transcription of Physicians' Orders. ❏

6. Record the medications in ink on the MAR under the correct heading by:
   a. writing: (1) today's date; (2) the name of the medication; (3) the dosage; (4) the route of administration; (5) the qualifying phrase, if used; and (6) the time of administration (refer to Table 13–1 in *Health Unit Coordinating*, 5th edition). ❏

✱ INFORMATION ALERT!

Some health care facilities prefer that the nurse fill in the specific time of administration. The times may vary due to type of medication, patient's home schedule, or patient's feeding schedule.

---

   b. writing the symbol "m" in ink on the doctor's order sheet to indicate completion of this step of transcription ❏

7. Recheck each step for accuracy. ❏

8. Sign-off the orders to indicate completion of transcription. ❏

Place a check mark (✔) in the box below to indicate that you have completed Activity 13–1.

❏ Transcribe Standing Medication Orders   Date: _____

ACTIVITY 13-2

TRANSCRIBE STANDING PRN MEDICATION ORDERS

Materials Needed
Black ink pen
Red ink pen (depending on hospital policy)
Pharmacy copy of the doctors' orders
PDR or pharmacology reference
MAR used in Activity 13–1
Computer and Practice Activity Software for Transcription of Physicians' Orders

Directions

Refer to Physicians' Order Sheet 13–2 in your patient's chart. Practice transcribing the standing prn medication orders by following the steps below. Check with your instructor for variations of this procedure to adapt it to the practice in your area. Place a check mark (✓) in the box as you complete each step.

Steps for Transcribing Standing PRN Medication Orders

1. Read the orders. ❏

2. Obtain the MAR. ❏

3. Order medications by faxing or sending the pharmacy copy of the doctor's orders to the pharmacy. ❏

4. Write "faxed" or "pcs" (pharmacy copy sent) with time and your initials in ink on the doctor's order sheet to indicate that the pharmacy copy has been sent. ❏

5. Enter medications on your patient's medication profile using a computer and the Practice Activity Software for the Transcription of Physicians' Orders. ❏

6. Record the medications in ink on the MAR under the correct heading by:
   a. writing (1) today's date; (2) the name of the medication; (3) the dosage; (4) the route of administration; (5) the qualifying phrase, if used; and (6) the time and date of administration ❏
   b. writing the symbol "m" in ink on the doctor's order sheet to indicate completion of this step of transcription ❏

7. Recheck each step for accuracy. ❏

8. Sign-off the orders to indicate completion of transcription. ❏

Place a check mark (✓) in the box below to indicate that you have completed Activity 13–2.

❏ Transcribe Standing PRN Medication Orders   Date: _____

ACTIVITY 13-3

TRANSCRIBE ONE-TIME MEDICATION ORDERS

Materials Needed   Black ink pen

Red ink pen (depending on hospital policy)

Pharmacy copy of doctors' orders

PDR or pharmacology reference

MAR used in Activity 13–2

Computer and Practice Activity Software for Transcription of Physicians' Orders

Directions

Refer to Physicians' Order Sheet 13–3 in your patient's chart. Practice transcribing the one-time medication orders by following the steps below. Check with your instructor for variations of the procedure to adapt it to the practice in your area. Place a check mark (✓) in the box as you complete each step.

Steps for Transcribing One-Time Medication Orders

1. Read the orders. ❏

2. Obtain the MAR. ❏

3. Order medications by faxing or sending the pharmacy copy of the doctor's orders to the pharmacy. ❏

4. Write "faxed" or "pcs" (pharmacy copy sent) with time and your initials in ink on the doctor's order sheet to indicate that the pharmacy copy has been sent. ❑

5. Enter medications on your patient's medication profile using a computer and the Practice Activity Software for Transcription of Physicians' Orders. ❑

6. Record the medications in ink on the MAR under the correct heading by:
   a. writing (1) today's date; (2) the name of the medication; (3) the dosage; (4) the route of administration; (5) the qualifying phrase, if used; and (6) the time and date of administration ❑
   b. writing the symbol "m" in ink on the doctor's order sheet to indicate completion of this step of transcription ❑

7. Recheck each step for accuracy. ❑

8. Sign-off the orders to indicate completion of transcription. ❑

Place a check mark (✔) in the box below to indicate that you have completed Activity 13–3.

❑ Transcribe One-Time Medication Orders   Date: _____

➤ **ACTIVITY 13-4**

TRANSCRIBE SHORT-ORDER SERIES MEDICATION ORDERS

Materials Needed   Black ink pen
Red ink pen (depending on hospital policy)
Pharmacy copy of the doctor's orders
PDR or pharmacology reference
Medication time schedule (Table 13–1) in *Health Unit Coordinating*, 5th edition.
MAR used in Activity 13–3
Computer and Practice Activity Software for Transcription of Physicians' Orders

Directions

Refer to Physicians' Order Sheet 13–4 on your patient's chart. Practice transcribing the short-order medication orders by following the steps below. Check with your instructor for variations of the procedure to adapt it to the practice in your area. Place a check mark (✔) in the box as you complete each step.

Steps for Transcribing Short-Order Medication Orders

1. Read the orders. ❑

2. Obtain medication records. ❑

3. Order medications by faxing or sending the pharmacy copy of the doctor's orders to the pharmacy. ❑

4. Write "faxed" or "pcs" (pharmacy copy sent) with time and your initials in ink on the doctor's order sheet to indicate that the pharmacy copy has been sent. ❑

5. Enter medications on your patient's medication profile using a computer and the Practice Activity Software for Transcription of Physicians' Orders. ❑

6. Record the medications in ink on the MAR under the correct heading by:
   a. writing (1) today's date; (2) the name of the medication; (3) the dosage; (4) the route of administration; (5) the qualifying phrase, if used; and (6) the time and date of administration ❑
   b. writing the symbol "m" in ink on the doctor's order sheet to indicate completion of this step of transcription ❑

7. Recheck each step for accuracy. ❑

8. Sign-off the orders to indicate completion of transcription. ❑

Place a check mark (✔) in the box below to indicate that you have completed Activity 13–4.

❑ Transcribe Short-Order Medication Orders   Date: _____

➤ ### ACTIVITY 13-5

TRANSCRIBE STAT MEDICATION ORDERS

Materials Needed   Black ink pen

Red ink pen (depending on hospital policy)

Pharmacy copy of the doctors' orders

PDR or pharmacology reference

MAR used in Activity 13–4

Computer and Practice Activity Software for Transcription of Physicians' Orders

Directions

Refer to Physicians' Order Sheet 13–5 in your patient's chart. Practice transcribing the stat medication orders by following the steps below. Check with your instructor for variations of the procedure to adapt it to the practice in your area. Place a check mark (✔) in the box as you complete each step.

Steps for Transcribing Stat Medication Orders

1. Read the orders. ❑

✱ INFORMATION ALERT!

In the hospital setting, communicate a stat medication order at once by notifying the nurse responsible for administering the medication to the patient. Note "name of nurse notified" with time and your initials on order sheet.

2. Notify the appropriate nurse and note "nurse notified" with time above the stat order. ❑

3. Obtain the MAR.

4. Order medications by faxing or sending the pharmacy copy of the doctor's orders to the pharmacy. ❑

5. Write "faxed" or "pcs" (pharmacy copy sent) with time and your initials in ink on the doctor's order sheet to indicate that the pharmacy copy has been sent. ❑

6. Enter medications on your patient's medication profile using a computer and the Practice Activity Software for Transcription of Physicians' Orders. ❑

7. Record the medications in ink on the MAR under the correct heading by:
   a. writing (1) today's date; (2) the name of the medication; (3) the dosage; (4) the route of administration. ❑
   b. writing the symbol "m" in ink on the doctor's order sheet to indicate completion of this step of transcription. ❑

8. Recheck each step for accuracy. ❑

9. Sign-off the orders to indicate completion of transcription. ❑

Place a check mark (✔) in the box below to indicate that you have completed Activity 13–5.

☐ Transcribe Stat Medication Orders   Date: _____

ACTIVITY 13-6

TRANSCRIBE MEDICATION ORDERS WITH AUTOMATIC STOP DATES

Materials Needed   Black ink pen
Red ink pen (depending on hospital policy)
Pharmacy copy of doctors' orders
PDR or pharmacology reference
Medication time schedule (Table 13–1 in *Health Unit Coordinating*, 5th ed.)
MAR used in Activity 13–5
Computer and Practice Activity Software for Transcription of Physicians' Orders

Directions

Refer to Physicians' Order Sheet 13–6 in your patient's chart. Practice transcribing the medication orders by following the steps below. Check with your instructor for variations of the procedure to adapt it to the practice in your area. Place a check mark (✔) in the box as you complete each step.

Steps for Transcribing Medication Orders with Automatic Stop Dates

1. Read the orders.   ☐

2. Obtain the MAR.   ☐

3. Order medications by faxing or sending the pharmacy copy of the doctor's orders to the pharmacy.   ☐

4. Write "faxed" or "pcs" (pharmacy copy sent) with time and your initials in ink
on the doctor's order sheet to indicate that the pharmacy copy has been sent.   ☐

✱ INFORMATION ALERT!

Medications such as narcotics, sedatives, antibiotics, and anticoagulants have automatic stop dates; that is, the physician will either reorder the medication or discontinue it by indicating his or her choice on a stamped or written request on the physician's order sheet. (The health unit coordinator or the nurse is responsible for placing this request on the order sheet.) Check with your instructor for the medications that have automatic stop dates in your area.

5. Enter medications on your patient's medication profile using a computer and the Practice
Activity Software for Transcription of Physicians' Orders.   ☐

6. Record the medications in ink on the MAR under the correct heading by:
a. writing (1) today's date; (2) the name of the medication; (3) the dosage; (4) the route of
administration; (5) the qualifying phrase, if used; (6) the time and date of administration
(for standing orders only); and the stop date in the stop date column next to the medication   ☐

> **✱ INFORMATION ALERT!**
>
> If two doses are included in one medication order, the doses must be written on separate lines on the medication record.
>
> **Example:**
>
> Percodan ī or ī̄ PO q 3–4 h prn
>
> | Date | Date | Dose | Route | Schedule |
> |------|------|------|-------|----------|
> | 0/00 | Percodan | ī | PO | q 3–4 h prn |
> | 0/00 | Percodan | ī̄ | PO | q 3–4 h prn |

    b. writing the symbol "m" in ink on the doctor's order sheet to indicate completion of this step of transcription ☐

7. Recheck each step for accuracy. ☐

8. Sign-off the orders to indicate completion of transcription. ☐

Place a check mark (✔) in the box below to indicate that you have completed Activity 13–6.

☐ Transcribe Medication Orders with Automatic Stop Dates   Date: _____

ACTIVITY 13-7

TRANSCRIBE IV MEDICATION ORDERS

Materials Needed

Black ink pen

Red ink pen (depending on hospital policy)

Pharmacy copy of doctor's orders

PDR or pharmacology reference

Medication time schedule (Table 13–1) in *Health Unit Coordinating,* 5th ed.

MAR used in Activity 13–6

Computer and Practice Activity Software for Transcription of Physicians' Orders

Directions

Refer to Physicians' Order Sheet 13–7 in your patient's chart. Practice transcribing the IV medication orders by following the steps below. Check with your instructor for variations of the procedure to adapt it to the practice in your area. Place a check mark (✓) in the box as you complete each step.

Steps for Transcribing IV Medication Orders

1. Read the orders. ☐

2. Obtain MAR. ☐

3. Order medications by faxing or sending the pharmacy copy of the doctor's orders to the pharmacy. ☐

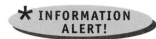

★ INFORMATION ALERT!

An admixture is a medication added to 500 to 1000 mL of IV solution; a piggyback medication is one added to 50 to 100 mL of IV solution. A bolus or IV push is a medication administered intravenously but not added to an IV solution.

4. Write "faxed" or "pcs" (pharmacy copy sent) with time and your initials in ink on the doctor's order sheet to indicate that the pharmacy copy has been sent. ❑

5. Enter medications on your patient's medication profile using a computer and the Practice Activity Software for Transcription of Physicians' Orders. ❑

6. Record the medications in ink on the MAR under the correct heading by:
   a. writing (1) today's date; (2) the name of the medication; (3) the dosage; (4) the route of administration; (5) the qualifying phrase, if used; (6) the time and date of administration; and (7) the stop date, if necessary ❑

★ INFORMATION ALERT!

In transcribing admixture orders, practice varies regarding whether the IV solution is recorded on the MAR.

   b. writing the symbol "m" in ink on the doctor's order sheet to indicate completion of this step of transcription ❑

7. Recheck each step for accuracy. ❑

8. Sign-off the orders to indicate completion of transcription. ❑

Place a check mark (✔) in the box below to indicate that you have completed Activity 13–7.

❑ Transcribe IV Medication Orders   Date: _____

ACTIVITY 13-8

TRANSCRIBE ORDERS TO RENEW MEDICATIONS THAT HAVE AUTOMATIC STOP DATES

Materials Needed   Black ink pen
Red ink pen (depending on hospital policy)
Pharmacy copy of the doctor's orders
PDR or pharmacology reference
MAR used in Activity 13–7
Computer and Practice Activity Software for Transcription of Physicians' Orders

Directions

Refer to Physicians' Order Sheet 13–8 in your patient's chart. Practice transcribing the orders to renew the medications by following the steps below. Check with your instructor for variations of the procedure to adapt it to the practice in your area. Place a check mark (✔) in the box as you complete each step.

Steps for Transcribing Orders to Renew Medications that Have Automatic Stop Dates

1. Read the orders. ☐

2. Obtain the MAR. ☐

3. Notify the pharmacy department that the medication(s) have been renewed by:
   a. faxing or sending the pharmacy copy of the doctor's order sheet to the pharmacy
   b. writing "faxed" or "pcs" (pharmacy copy sent) with time and your initials in ink on
      the doctor's order sheet to indicate that the pharmacy copy has been sent ☐

4. Enter the new stop dates on your patient's medication profile by using a computer and
   the Practice Activity Software for Transcription of Physicians' Orders ☐

5. Renew the medications on the MAR by:
   a. placing a slash mark across the stop date in the stop date column ☐
   b. writing the new stop date in ink near the stop date column next to the medication ☐

✱ INFORMATION ALERT!

Method of renewing medication on the MAR may vary among hospitals. In some hospitals, the stop date is written in pencil and is erased and new stop date entered (the original order date remains and is written in ink).

   c. writing the symbol "m" in ink on the doctor's order sheet to indicate completion of
      this step of transaction ☐

6. Recheck each step for accuracy. ☐

7. Sign-off the order to indicate completion of transcription. ☐

Place a check mark (✔) in the box below to indicate that you have completed Activity 13–8.

☐ Transcribe Orders to Renew Medications that Have
   Automatic Stop Dates   Date: _____

ACTIVITY 13-9

TRANSCRIBE ORDERS TO DISCONTINUE MEDICATIONS

Materials Needed   Black ink pen
                          Red ink pen (depending on hospital policy)
                          Yellow highlighter
                          Pharmacy copy of doctors' orders
                          MAR used in Activity 13–8
                          Computer and Practice Activity Software for Transcription of Physicians' Orders

Directions

Refer to Physicians' Order Sheet 13–9 in your patient's chart. Practice transcribing orders to discontinue the medications by following the steps below. Check with your instructor for variations of the procedure to adapt it to the practice in your area. Place a check mark (✔) in the box as you complete each step.

Steps for Transcribing Orders to Discontinue Medications

1. Read the orders. ☐

2. Obtain the MAR. ☐

3. Notify the pharmacy department that the medication(s) have been discontinued by:
   a. faxing or sending the pharmacy copy of the doctor's order sheet to the pharmacy ❏
   b. Writing "faxed" or "pcs" (pharmacy copy sent) with time and your initials in ink on the doctor's order sheet to indicate that the pharmacy copy has been sent. ❏

4. Discontinue the medications on your patient's medication profile by typing "DC'd" next to the medication using a computer and the Practice Activity Software for Transcription of Physicians' Orders. ❏

5. Discontinue the medications on the MAR by:
   a. highlighting the medication and all spaces on the line of the discontinued medication using a yellow highlighter ❏
   b. recording "D/C" in ink on the line of the discontinued medication under the correct date ❏
   c. writing the symbol "m" in ink on the doctor's order sheet to indicate completion of this step of transaction ❏

6. Recheck each step for accuracy. ❏

7. Sign-off the orders to indicate completion of transcription. ❏

Place a check mark (✔) in the box below to indicate that you have completed Activity 13–9.

❏ Transcribe Orders to Discontinue Medications   Date: _____

ACTIVITY 13-10

TRANSCRIBE ORDERS FOR MEDICATION CHANGES

Materials Needed   Black ink pen
Red ink pen (depending on hospital policy)
Yellow highlighter
Pharmacy copy of doctors' orders
Medication time schedule (Table 13–1) in *Health Unit Coordinating*, 5th ed.
MAR used in Activity 13–9
Computer and Practice Activity Software for Transcription of Physicians' Orders

Directions

Refer to Physicians' Order Sheet 13–10 in your patient's chart. Practice transcribing the orders for the medication changes by following the steps below. Check with your instructor for variations of the procedure to adapt it to the practice in your area. Place a check mark (✔) in the box as you complete each step.

Steps for Transcribing Orders for Medication Changes

1. Read the orders. ❏

2. Obtain the MAR. ❏

3. Notify the pharmacy department that the medication(s) has (have) been changed by:
   a. faxing or sending the pharmacy copy of the doctor's order sheet to the pharmacy ❏
   b. writing "faxed" or "pcs" (pharmacy copy sent) with time and your initials in ink on the doctor's order sheet to indicate that the pharmacy copy has been sent ❏

4. Record the medication change on your patient's medication profile by typing "DC'd" next to the discontinued medication and then typing the correct medication on the next line, using a computer and the Practice Activity Software for Transcription of Physicians' Orders. ❏

5. Record the medication changes on the MAR by:
   a. highlighting the original order and the unused spaces using the yellow highlighter ☐
   b. writing "D/C" or Δ on the line of the discontinued (changed) medication under the correct date in ink ☐
   c. writing in the new order on a new line ☐
   d. writing the symbol "m" in ink on the doctor's order sheet to indicate completion
     of this step of transaction ☐

6. Recheck each step for accuracy. ☐

7. Sign-off the orders to indicate completion of transcription. ☐

Place a check mark (✔) in the box below to indicate that you have completed Activity 13–10.

☐ Transcribe Orders for Medication Changes   Date: _____

ACTIVITY 13-11

TRANSCRIBE A REVIEW SET OF MEDICATION ORDERS

Materials Needed   Black ink pen
                             Red ink pen (depending on hospital policy)
                             Yellow highlighter
                             Pharmacy copy of the doctor's orders
                             PDR or pharmacology reference
                             Medication time schedule (Table 13–1) in *Health Unit Coordinating*, 5th ed.
                             MAR used in Activity 13–10
                             Computer and Practice Activity Software for Transcription of Physicians' Orders

Directions

Refer to Physicians' Order Sheet 13–11 in your patient's chart. Transcribe the orders. They include changing, renewing, and discontinuing medication orders. Refer to previous medication activities for the appropriate transcription steps as needed.

Steps for Transcribing a Review Set of Medication Orders

1. Read the orders. ☐

2. Order medications by faxing or sending the pharmacy copy of the doctors' orders
to the pharmacy and write "faxed" or "pcs" (pharmacy copy sent) with time and
your initials in ink on doctor's order sheet. ☐

3. Check for any stat orders. ☐

4. Obtain the MAR. ☐

5. Order any supplies needed. ☐

6. Enter the medications on your patient's medication profile by using a computer
and the Practice Activity Software for Transcription of Physicians' Orders. ☐

7. Record the medications on the MAR. ☐

8. Recheck each step for accuracy. ☐

9. Sign-off the orders to indicate completion of transcription. ☐

Place a check mark (✓) in the box below to indicate that you have completed Activity 13–11.

☐ Transcribe a Review Set of Medication Orders   Date: _____

★ **INFORMATION ALERT!**

Many health care facility pharmacies have a computer system that will generate a printed copy of each patient's prescribed medications each morning. Additions, deletions, and changes will be written in during the day. Pharmacy copies or faxed physician's order sheets will notify the pharmacy department of changes so the printed list for the next day will reflect changes.

➤ **ACTIVITY 13-12**

TRANSCRIBE A REVIEW SET OF DOCTORS' ORDERS

Materials Needed

Black ink pen
Red ink pen (depending on hospital policy)
Pencil
Eraser
Patient's ID labels (if using requisition method)
Necessary requisitions (if using requisition method)
PDR or pharmacology reference
Medication time schedule (Table 13–1) in *Health Unit Coordinating*, 4th ed.
Kardex used in previous chapters
MAR used in Activity 13–11
Computer and Practice Activity Software for Transcription of Physicians' Orders

Directions

Refer to Physicians' Order Sheet 13–12 in your patient's chart. Transcribe the orders. Refer to the previous activities for the appropriate transcription steps as needed.

Steps for Transcribing a Review Set of Doctors' Orders

1. Read the orders.   ☐
2. Order medications by faxing or sending the pharmacy copy of the doctors' orders to the pharmacy and write "faxed" or "pcs" (pharmacy copy sent) with time and your initials in ink on doctor's order sheet.   ☐
3. Check for any stat orders.   ☐
4. Make any necessary phone calls.   ☐
5. Obtain the necessary forms.   ☐

Suggestion to the student: Use this space to list the forms you will need.

6. Order as necessary. ❑

7. Kardex the orders. ❑

8. Enter the medications on your patient's medication profile by using a computer and the Practice Activity Software for Transcription of Physicians' Orders. ❑

9. Record the medications on the MAR. ❑

10. Recheck each step for accuracy. ❑

11. Sign-off the orders to indicate completion of transcription. ❑

✱ INFORMATION ALERT!

Transcribing doctors' orders is a critical task, and an error could cause harm to a patient. If you are not absolutely sure of what the medication is or have any doubt about an order, ask the patient's nurse or the doctor who wrote the order.

Place a check mark (✔) in the box below to indicate that you have completed Activity 13–12.

❑ Transcribe a Review Set of Doctors' Orders   Date: _____

ACTIVITY 13-13

LOCATE MEDICATIONS IN THE *PHYSICIANS' DESK REFERENCE*

Materials Needed   Pen or pencil

Physicians' Desk Reference (PDR)

Paper

Directions

Locate the following medications in the PDR using the section titled "Brand and Generic Name Index," and briefly state the purpose of each. (Read the paragraph[s] titled "Indications and Usage" under the drug name in the "Product Information" section to locate the purpose.) Your instructor may ask you to locate and record additional information. Follow the steps below. Place a check mark (✓) in the box as you complete each step.

Medications

Demerol	Lanoxin
Synthroid	Zantac
Klor-Con	Lasix
amoxicillin	heparin
Ceclor	Dilantin

Steps for Locating Medications in the Physicians' Desk Reference

1. Locate the medication (listed alphabetically) in the "Generic and Brand Name Index" (pink section) of the PDR. ☐

2. Turn to the page (higher number) indicated next to the medication. ☐

3. Read the paragraph(s) titled "Indications and Usage" under drug name and record the purpose of the medication. ☐

Place a check mark (✔) in the box below to indicate that you have completed Activity 13–13.

☐ Locate Medications in the *Physician's Desk Reference*　　Date: _____

ACTIVITY 13-14

RECORD TELEPHONED DOCTORS' ORDERS

Materials Needed　Pen
　　　　　　　　　　Physician's order sheet

Directions

Practice recording the telephoned doctor's orders printed below by following the steps below. Place a check mark (✓) in the box as you complete each step.

Telephoned Doctors' Orders

"Hello, this is Dr. Browning with some orders on Penny Pincher.

Start intravenous fluids of 1000 ccs of lactated Ringer's with 40 milliequivalents potassium chloride to run at 125 cubic centimeters per hour
Ampicillin 250 milligrams intravenous piggyback every 8 hours
Torecan suppository every 4 hours for nausea and vomiting
Lomotil one tablet orally after each loose stool
Demerol 50 or 100 milligrams every 3 or 4 hours for pain
Tylenol suppository grain ten every 3 hours for temperature over 102 degrees per rectum

Have Penny's nurse call me with the morning vital signs and an update on Penny's condition. Thanks."

Steps for Recording Telephoned Doctors' Orders

1. Have someone read the above orders to you while you record them on a physician's order sheet. ☐

2. Use accepted abbreviations and symbols as you write the orders. ☐

3. Follow the guidelines you have written in Activity 9–1. ☐

4. For further practice, obtain a new Kardex form and practice transcribing the orders you have written. ☐

Place a check mark (✔) in the box below to indicate that you have completed Activity 13–14.

☐ Record Telephoned Doctors' Orders   Date: _____

ACTIVITY 13-15

RECORD TELEPHONE MESSAGES

Materials Needed   Pen or pencil
                           Message pad

Directions

Practice recording the telephone messages printed below by following the steps below. Place a check mark (✔) in the box as you complete each step.

Telephone Messages

1. "This is Dr. Joan Peters. Would you let Fanny Pack's nurse know that I will be in to write total parenteral nutrition orders in about a half an hour?"

2. "This is Dave in the pharmacy. I received a pharmacy copy that was not labeled with a patient's name. I am sending it back to you to identify, label, and send back to me."

Steps for Recording Telephone Messages

1. Have someone read the above messages to you while you record them on a message pad.   ☐

2. Write down for whom the message is intended.   ☐

3. Write down the caller's name.   ☐

4. Write down the date and time of the call.   ☐

5. Write down the purpose of the call.   ☐

6. If a return call is expected, write down the number to call.   ☐

7. Sign your name to the message.   ☐

Place a check mark (✔) in the box below to indicate that you have completed Activity 13–15.

☐ Record Telephone Messages   Date: _____

PHYSICIANS' ORDER SHEET 13–1

DATE	TIME	SYMBOL	ORDERS
			Xanax .05 mg PO qid
			Amoxicillin 500 mg PO q 8°
			Anusol HC supp q hs
			Lanoxin 0.25 mg PO qd
			Neosporin ung ophthalmic OD bid
			Vit B$_{12}$ 100 mcg IM qod
			Dr

PHYSICIANS' ORDER SHEET 13–2

DATE	TIME	SYMBOL	ORDERS
			Antivert 25 mg PO q 24 hr as needed
			Tylenol 650 mg PO q 4 hr for H/A
			Compazine supp 5 mg prn N/V
			Ativan 1 mg PO q 3 hr prn for restlessness
			Dr

PHYSICIANS' ORDER SHEET 13–3

DATE	TIME	SYMBOL	ORDERS
			Clarinex 2.5 mg PO this AM—may repeat this PM if nec
			Demerol 100 mg IM tomorrow @ 0800 ā abd dressing △
			Dr
			PPD ID today
			Dr

PHYSICIANS' ORDER SHEET 13–4

DATE	TIME	SYMBOL	ORDERS
			Kaon 15 ml in $^1/_2$ glass H$_2$O c̄ meals x 3 days
			Aquamephyton 10 mg IM daily x 3
			Lasix 40 mg PO today, then 20 mg qd x 3
			Imodium 4 mg this AM, then 2 mg PO p̄ ea unformed
			stool (maximum 6 mg)
			Dr

PHYSICIANS' ORDER SHEET 13–5

DATE	TIME	SYMBOL	ORDERS
			Heparin 20,000 U IV push stat
			Librium 10 mg PO stat
			Compazine 10 mg IM now
			Dr

PHYSICIANS' ORDER SHEET 13–6

DATE	TIME	SYMBOL	ORDERS
			Restoril 15 mg PO q hs
			Percocet 1 or 2 tabs q 3-4 hr prn for moderate pain
			Lovenox 40 mg sq qd
			Dr
			MS 10 mg q 3-4 hr prn severe pain
			Dr

PHYSICIANS' ORDER SHEET 13–7

DATE	TIME	SYMBOL	ORDERS
			Zinacef 750 mg IVPB q 8° x 2 doses
			Compazine 5 mg IV q 4 hr for N/V
			Start IV of 1000 cc LR c̄ 1 amp MVI 100 cc/hr—call
			hospitalist if IV infiltrates
			Dr

PHYSICIANS' ORDER SHEET 13–8

DATE	TIME	SYMBOL	ORDERS
			Renew
			Restoril 15 mg
			MS 10 mg
			Dr

PHYSICIANS' ORDER SHEET 13–9

DATE	TIME	SYMBOL	ORDERS
			D/C Xanax
			D/C Amoxicillin
			D/C Imodium
			Dr

PHYSICIANS' ORDER SHEET 13–10

DATE	TIME	SYMBOL	ORDERS
			△ Lanoxin to 0.125 mg daily
			△ Lovenox to 20 mg qd
			D/C Neosporin ung
			Dr

PHYSICIANS' ORDER SHEET 13–11

DATE	TIME	SYMBOL	ORDERS
			Lantus 18 u sq hs
			Albuterol ii puffs qid
			HCTZ 25 mg PO qd
			Synthroid 112 mcg qd
			Dr
			D/C anusol HC
			D/C compazine
			Phenergan 25 mg IV q 4° N/V
			Vancomycin 1 gm IVPB q 12 hr
			Flexeril 20 mg PO bid
			Dr
			D/C peripheral IV
			MVI tab i PO qd
			Atenolol 25 mg PO qd
			NTG $^{1}/_{150}$ subling. for chest pain @ bedside
			Dr

PHYSICIANS' ORDER SHEET 13–12

DATE	TIME	SYMBOL	ORDERS
			1200 cal ADA diet
			BR c̄ BSC
			VS q 4 hr—call if SBP ↑ 180 or ↓ 110
			ORE this AM
			D/C pneumatic hose
			D/C alternating pressure pad
			Monitor blood glucose AC & HS—sliding scale as follows:
			200-249 give 5 u regular insulin
			250-299 give 10 u regular insulin
			300-349 give 15 u regular insulin
			>349—call hospitalist
			Prednisone 20 mg PO bid x 7 days, then 10 mg x 5 days,
			then 5 mg qd
			D/C Flexeril
			Celebrex 400 mg PO bid c̄ food
			Timoptic ophthalmic solution 0.25% ī gtt .05 bid
			Monopril 10 mg PO q day
			D/C orthostatic BP's
			Insert foley cath
			Dr

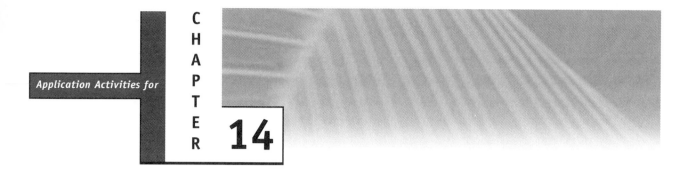

Laboratory Orders and Recording Telephoned Laboratory Results

Place the Physicians' Order Sheets located at the end of the chapter in your patient's chart. Follow the directions for each activity to transcribe orders.

Activities in This Chapter

ACTIVITY 14-1

TRANSCRIBE HEMATOLOGY/COAGULATION ORDERS

Materials Needed

Black ink pen

Red ink pen (depending on hospital policy)

Pencil

Eraser

Kardex form used in previous chapters

Patient ID labels (if using requisition method)

Laboratory requisition form (if using requisition method)

Computer and Practice Activity Software for Transcription of Physicians' Orders

Directions

Refer to Physicians' Order Sheet 14–1 in your patient's chart. Practice transcribing the hematology/coagulation orders by following the steps below. Check with your instructor for variations of the procedure to adapt it to the practice in your area. Place a check mark (✓) in the box as you complete each step.

Steps for Transcribing Hematology/Coagulation Orders

1. Read the orders. ☐

2. Obtain the Kardex form and requisition form if using the requisition method. ☐

3. Order the test(s) from the laboratory department.

Use the computer method by:

a. selecting Enter Orders on the master screen

b. selecting the patient's name from the census on the viewing screen ☐

c. selecting the laboratory department from the department menu on the viewing screen ☐

d. selecting the hematology division from the laboratory department viewing screen ☐

e. typing in the pertinent information ☐

f. selecting the test(s) to be ordered from the menu on the viewing screen ☐

g. writing "ord" in ink above each order on the doctors' order sheet to indicate that the test has been ordered ☐

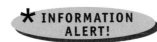

★ INFORMATION ALERT!

In the hospital setting, writing "ord" or the computer order number above each laboratory test ordered will reduce the risk of missing an order.

h. sending the order by pressing "enter" on the computer keyboard ☐

Use the requisition method by:

a. labeling the laboratory requisition with the patient's ID label ☐

b. writing in the pertinent information ☐

c. placing a check mark (✓) in the column next to the test(s) to be ordered ☐

d. writing "ord" in ink above each order on the doctors' order sheet to indicate that the test has been ordered ☐

e. sending the requisition ☐

4. Kardex the orders by:

a. writing the date and the order in pencil in the lab column on the Kardex form ☐

b. writing the symbol "K" in ink in front of the order on the doctors' order sheet to indicate completion of the kardexing step ☐

5. Recheck each step for accuracy. ☐

6. Sign off the orders to indicate completion of transcription. ☐

Place a check mark (✔) in the box below to indicate that you have completed Activity 14–1.

☐ Transcribe Hematology/Coagulation Orders   Date: _____

ACTIVITY 14-2

TRANSCRIBE DAILY LABORATORY ORDERS

Materials Needed   Black ink pen

Red ink pen (depending on hospital policy)

Pencil

Eraser

Kardex form used in Activity 14–1

Patient ID labels (if using requisition method)

Laboratory requisition (if using requisition method)

Computer and Practice Activity Software for Transcription of Physicians' Orders

Directions

Refer to Physicians' Order Sheet 14–2 in your patient's chart. Practice transcribing the daily laboratory orders by following the steps below. Check with your instructor for variations of the procedure to adapt it to the practice in your area. Place a check mark (✓) in the box as you complete each step.

Steps for transcribing daily laboratory orders

1. Read the orders. ☐

2. Obtain the Kardex form and requisition form if using the requisition method. ☐

3. Order the test(s) from the laboratory department.

Use the computer method by:
a. selecting Enter Orders on the master screen
b. selecting the patient's name from the census on the viewing screen ☐
c. selecting the laboratory department from the department menu on the viewing screen ☐
d. selecting the hematology division from the laboratory department viewing screen ☐
e. typing in the pertinent information ☐
f. selecting the test(s) to be ordered from the menu on the viewing screen ☐
g. writing "ord" in ink above each order on the doctors' order sheet to indicate that the test has been ordered ☐
h. sending the order by pressing "enter" on the computer keyboard ☐

Use the requisition method by:
a. labeling the laboratory requisition with patient ID label ☐
b. writing in the pertinent information ☐
c. placing a check mark (✓) in the column next to the test(s) to be ordered ☐
d. writing "ord" in ink above each order on the doctors' order sheet to indicate that the test has been ordered ☐
e. sending the requisition ☐

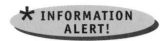

The date and time that the daily laboratory tests will be drawn vary according to hospital policy. Most daily lab tests are ordered to be done at 0400 so the physicians may have the results when they make rounds on their patients. Check with your instructor for the practice in your area.

4. Kardex the orders by:
  a. writing the date and the order in pencil in the daily lab column on the Kardex form ❑
  b. writing the symbol "K" in ink in front of the order on the doctors' order sheet to indicate completion of the kardexing step ❑
5. Recheck each step for accuracy. ❑
6. Sign off the orders to indicate completion of transcription. ❑

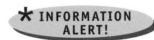

Daily laboratory tests may be ordered from all divisions of the laboratory. Most computer systems have the capacity to order daily diagnostic tests for several days in advance. If not, the daily order must be entered each day for the following day.

Place a check mark (✔) in the box below to indicate that you have completed Activity 14–2.

❑ Transcribe Daily Laboratory Orders   Date: _____

ACTIVITY 14-3

TRANSCRIBE CHEMISTRY ORDERS

Materials Needed   Black ink pen
                         Red ink pen (depending on hospital policy)
                         Pencil
                         Eraser
                         Kardex form used in Activity 14–2
                         Patient ID labels (if using requisition method)
                         Laboratory requisition (if using requisition method)
                         Computer and Practice Activity Software for Transcription of Physicians' Orders

Directions

Refer to Physicians' Order Sheet 14–3 in your patient's chart. Practice transcribing the chemistry orders following the steps below. Check with your instructor for variations of the procedure to adapt it to the practice in your area. Place a check mark (✔) in the box as you complete each step.

Steps for Transcribing Chemistry Orders

1. Read the orders. ❑

2. Obtain the Kardex form and requisition form if using the requisition method. ❑

3. Order the test(s) from the laboratory department. ❑

Use the computer method by:
a. selecting Enter Orders from the master screen
b. selecting the patient's name from the census on the viewing screen ❑
c. selecting the laboratory department from the department menu on the viewing screen ❑
d. selecting the chemistry division from the laboratory department viewing screen ❑
e. typing in the pertinent information ❑
f. selecting the test(s) to be ordered from the menu on the viewing screen ❑
g. writing "ord" in ink above the order on the doctors' order sheet to indicate that the test has been ordered ❑
h. sending the order by pressing "enter" on the computer keyboard ❑

Use the requisition method by:
a. labeling with patient ID label ❑
b. writing in the pertinent information ❑
c. placing a check mark (✓) in the column next to the test(s) to be ordered ❑
d. writing "ord" in ink above each order on the doctors' order sheet to indicate that the test has been ordered ❑
e. sending the requisition ❑

4. Kardex the orders by:
a. writing the date and the order in pencil in the lab column on the Kardex form ❑
b. writing the symbol "K" in ink in front of the order on the doctors' order sheet to indicate completion of the kardexing step ❑

5. Recheck each step for accuracy. ❑

6. Sign off the orders to indicate completion of transcription. ❑

Place a check mark (✔) in the box below to indicate that you have completed Activity 14–3.

❑ Transcribe Chemistry Orders   Date: _____

ACTIVITY 14-4

TRANSCRIBE STAT LABORATORY ORDERS

Materials Needed

Black ink pen

Red ink pen (depending on hospital policy)

Pencil

Eraser

Kardex form used in Activity 14–3

Patient ID labels (if using requisition method)

Laboratory (if using requisition method)

Computer and Practice Activity Software for Transcription of Physicians' Orders

Directions

Refer to Physicians' Order Sheet 14–4 in your patient's chart. Practice transcribing the stat laboratory orders by following the steps below. Check with your instructor for variations of the procedure to adapt it to the practice in your area. Place a check mark (✓) in the box as you complete each step.

Steps for Transcribing Stat Laboratory Orders

1. Read the orders. ❑

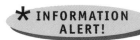

> Communicate stat laboratory orders by immediately notifying the laboratory or nursing personnel responsible for carrying out the order. Include the name of the patient, the room number, and the test requested (if nursing personnel will be drawing lab, supply with copy of order). Record the word "notified" and time you notified the laboratory or nursing personnel next to the stat order on the doctors' order sheet. Stat orders communicated by computer may not require a telephone call to laboratory personnel. Enter "stat" under the pertinent information heading on computer requisition.

2. Obtain the Kardex form and requisition form if using the requisition method. ❑

3. Order the tests(s) from the laboratory department. ❑

Use the computer method by:
a. selecting Enter Orders from the master screen ❑
b. selecting the patient's name from the census on the viewing screen ❑
c. selecting the laboratory department from the department menu on the viewing screen ❑
d. selecting the appropriate division from the laboratory department viewing screen ❑
e. typing in the pertinent information (remember to select "stat" on the computer) ❑
f. selecting the test(s) to be ordered from the menu on the viewing screen ❑
g. writing "ord" in ink above each order on the doctors' order sheet to indicate that the test has been ordered ❑
h. sending the order by pressing "enter" on the computer keyboard ❑

Use the requisition method by:
a. labeling the laboratory requisition with patient ID label ❑
b. writing in the pertinent information ❑
c. placing a check mark (✓) in the column next to the test(s) to be ordered ❑
d. writing "ord" in ink above each order on the doctors' order sheet to indicate that the test has been ordered ❑
e. sending the requisition ❑

4. Kardex the orders by. ❑
a. writing the date and order in pencil in the lab column on the Kardex form ❑
b. writing the symbol "K" in ink in front of the order on the doctors' order sheet to indicate completion of the kardexing step ❑

5. Recheck each step for accuracy. ❑

6. Sign off the order to indicate completion of transcription. ❑

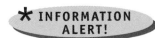

> Most health care facilities have a 1-hour time limit to draw stat labs and a 4-hour time limit to draw routine labs. Stat labs in life-threatening or code situations would be drawn immediately.

Place a check mark (✔) in the box below to indicate that you have completed Activity 14–4.

☐ Transcribe Stat Laboratory Orders   Date: _____

ACTIVITY 14-5

TRANSCRIBE FASTING AND NPO LABORATORY ORDERS

Materials Needed   Black ink pen

Red ink pen (depending on hospital policy)

Pencil

Eraser

Kardex form used in Activity 14–4

Patient ID labels (if using requisition method)

Laboratory requisition (if using requisition method)

Computer and Practice Activity Software for Transcription of Physicians' Orders

Fasting and/or NPO list for laboratory studies (Table 14–1) in *Health Unit Coordinating*, 5th edition, page 272.

Directions

Refer to Physicians' Order Sheet 14–5 in your patient's chart. Practice transcribing the fasting and NPO laboratory orders by following the steps below. Check with your instructor for variations of the procedure to adapt it to the practice in your area. Place a check mark (✔) in the box as you complete each step.

Steps for Transcribing Fasting and NPO Laboratory Orders

1. Read the orders.   ☐

2. Obtain the Kardex form and requisition form if using the requisition method.   ☐

3. Order the test(s) from the laboratory department.   ☐

Use the computer method by:
a. selecting Enter Order on the master screen
b. selecting the patient's name from the census on the viewing screen   ☐
c. selecting the laboratory department from the department menu on the viewing screen   ☐
d. selecting the chemistry division from the laboratory department viewing screen   ☐
e. typing in the pertinent information   ☐
f. selecting the test(s) to be ordered from the menu on the viewing screen   ☐
g. writing "ord" in ink above each order on the doctors' order sheet to indicate
   that the test has been ordered   ☐
h. sending the order by pressing "enter" on the computer keyboard   ☐

Use the requisition method by:
a. labeling the laboratory requisition with patient ID label   ☐
b. writing in the pertinent information   ☐
c. placing a check mark (✔) in the column next to the test(s) to be ordered   ☐
d. writing "ord" in ink above each order on the doctors' order sheet to indicate that the
   test has been ordered   ☐
e. sending the requisition   ☐

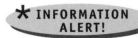

★ INFORMATION ALERT!

Select or enter the date and time the laboratory personnel should draw the blood when ordering a laboratory test on the computer. When using the requisition method, write the date and time to draw the blood at the top of the requisition. For fasting and NPO orders, the blood is drawn before breakfast the following day.

4. Kardex the orders by:
   a. writing the date and order in pencil in the lab column on the Kardex form ☐
   b. writing the symbol "K" in ink in front of the order on the doctors' order sheet to indicate completion of the kardexing step ☐

5. Recheck each step for accuracy. ☐

6. Sign off the orders to indicate completion of transcription. ☐

Place a check mark (✔) in the box below to indicate that you have completed Activity 14–5.

☐ Transcribe Fasting and NPO Laboratory Orders   Date: _____

 ACTIVITY 14-6

TRANSCRIBE A REVIEW SET OF LABORATORY ORDERS

Materials Needed

Black ink pen

Red ink pen (depending on hospital policy)

Pencil

Eraser

Kardex form used in Activity 14–5

Patient ID labels (if using requisition method)

Laboratory requisition (if using requisition method)

Computer and Practice Activity Software for Transcription of Physicians' Orders

Fasting and/or NPO lists for laboratory studies Table 14–1 in *Health Unit Coordinating*, 5th edition, page 272

Directions

Refer to Physicians' Order Sheet 14–6 in your patient's chart. Transcribe the orders. They include hematology/coagulation, daily lab studies, chemistry, toxicology, stat, and fasting and NPO laboratory orders. Refer to previous activities for the appropriate transcription steps as needed.

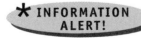

★ INFORMATION ALERT!

Peak-and-trough drug levels are ordered in the toxicology division of the laboratory and require the health unit coordinator to coordinate the ordering of the blood draws with the nurse administering the drug, such as vancomycin. The trough is ordered timed stat (T/stat), meaning that it will be drawn stat at the specific time indicated.

Steps for Transcribing a Review Set of Laboratory Orders

1. Read the orders.   ❑

2. Check orders for stats.   ❑

3. Obtain the Kardex form and requisition forms if using the requisition method.   ❑

4. Order the tests.   ❑

5. Kardex the orders.   ❑

6. Recheck each step for accuracy.   ❑

7. Sign off the orders to indicate completion of transcription.   ❑

Place a check mark (✔) in the box below to indicate that you have completed Activity 14–6.

❑ Transcribe a Review Set of Laboratory Orders   Date: _____

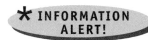

ACTIVITY 14-7

TRANSCRIBE MICROBIOLOGY/ BACTERIOLOGY ORDERS

Materials Needed   Black ink pen

Red ink pen (depending on hospital policy)

Pencil

Eraser

Kardex form used in Activity 14–6

Patient ID labels (if using requisition method)

Laboratory requisition (if using requisition method)

Computer and Practice Activity Software for Transcription of Physicians' Orders

Directions

Refer to Physicians' Order Sheet 14–7 in your patient's chart. Practice transcribing the microbiology/bacteriology orders by following the steps below. Check with your instructor for variations of the procedure to adapt it to the practice in your area. Place a check mark (✔) in the box as you complete each step.

✱ INFORMATION ALERT!

> Standard precautions require that all specimens be bagged and labeled with patient ID information. The date and time specimens were collected should be written on the patient ID label with initials of the person that collected the specimen. The person collecting the specimen should do this. In emergency situations, the health unit coordinator may need to label and bag specimens. Gloves should be kept in a drawer at the nursing station to wear when this happens and the health unit coordinator should always wash his/her hands after handling specimens bagged or not.

Steps for Transcribing Microbiology/Bacteriology Orders

1. Read the orders.   ❑

2. Obtain the Kardex form, requisition forms if using the requisition method, and patient ID labels.   ❑

3. Order the test(s) from the laboratory department.

Use the computer method by:
a. selecting Enter Orders on the master screen ❑
b. selecting the patient's name from the census on the viewing screen ❑
c. selecting the laboratory department from the department menu on the viewing screen ❑
d. selecting the microbiology division from the laboratory department viewing screen ❑
e. typing in the pertinent information ❑
f. selecting the specimen source from the menu on the viewing screen ❑
g. selecting the test(s) to be performed from the menu on the viewing screen ❑
h. writing "ord" in ink above each order on the doctor's order sheet to indicate that the test has been ordered ❑
i. when collected, look through bag that contains the specimen and check label on specimen for proper patient ID, date, and time collected and for initials of person who collected specimen ❑
j. sending the specimen with a copy of the order to the laboratory ❑

✱ INFORMATION ALERT!

The order is usually entered into the computer when the specimen is obtained. The bagged, labeled specimen is then sent to the laboratory with a copy of the computer requisition.

Use the requisition method by:
a. labeling the laboratory requisitions with patient ID labels ❑

✱ INFORMATION ALERT!

Most specimens obtained from the patient by the nurse require a separate requisition and label, because they may be collected at different times or sent to different divisions within the laboratory. In the hospital setting, the label is paper-clipped to the requisition and kept at the nursing unit in a designated area until the nurse obtains the specimen.

b. writing in the pertinent information ❑
c. placing a check mark (✓) in the column next to the test(s) to be ordered ❑
d. writing "ord" in ink above each order on the doctors' order sheet to indicate that the test has been ordered ❑
e. when collected, check label on specimen for proper patient ID, date, and time collected and for initials of person who collected specimen ❑
f. send the specimen with the requisition to the laboratory ❑

4. Kardex the orders by:
a. writing the date and the order in pencil in the lab column on the Kardex form ❑
b. writing the symbol "K" in ink in front of the order on the doctors' order sheet to indicate completion of the kardexing step ❑

5. Recheck each step for accuracy. ❑

6. Sign off the orders to indicate completion of transcription. ❑

Place a check mark (✔) in the box below to indicate that you have completed Activity 14–7.

❑ Transcribe Microbiology/Bacteriology Orders   Date: _____

ACTIVITY 14-8

TRANSCRIBE SEROLOGY ORDERS

Materials Needed   Black ink pen
Red ink pen (depending on hospital policy)
Pencil
Eraser
Kardex form used in Activity 14–7
Patient ID labels (if using requisition method)
Laboratory requisition (if using requisition method)
Computer and Practice Activity Sofware for Transcription of Physicians' Orders

Directions

Refer to Physicians' Order Sheet Fig. 14–8 in your patient's chart. Practice transcribing the serology orders by following the steps below. Check with your instructor for variations of the procedure to adapt it to the practice in your area. Place a check mark (✓) in the box as you complete each step.

Steps for Transcribing Serology Orders

1. Read the orders. ❑

2. Obtain the Kardex form and requisition form if using the requisition method. ❑

3. Order the test(s) from the laboratory department.

Use the computer method by:
a   selecting *Enter Orders* on the master screen
b. selecting the patient's name from the census on the viewing screen ❑
c. selecting the laboratory department from the department menu on the viewing screen ❑
d. selecting the serology division from the laboratory department viewing screen ❑
e. typing in the pertinent information ❑
f.   selecting the test(s) to be ordered from the menu on the viewing screen ❑
g. writing "ord" or the computer order number in ink above each order on the doctors'
order sheet to indicate that the test has been ordered ❑
h. sending the order by pressing "enter" on the computer keyboard ❑

Use the requisition method by:
a. labeling the laboratory requisition with patient ID label ❑
b. writing in the pertinent information ❑
c. placing a check mark (✓) in the column next to the test(s) to be ordered ❑
d. writing "ord" in ink above each order on the doctors' order sheet to indicate that the
test has been ordered ❑
e. sending the requisition ❑

4. Kardex the orders by:
a. writing the date and the order in pencil in the lab column on the Kardex form ❑
b. writing the symbol "K" in ink in front of the order on the doctors' order sheet to indicate
completion of the kardexing step ❑

5. Recheck each step for accuracy. ❑

6. Sign off the order to indicate completion of transcription. ❑

Place a check mark (✔) in the box below to indicate that you have completed Activity 14–8.

❑ Transcribe Serology Orders   Date: _____

ACTIVITY 14-9

TRANSCRIBE A BLOOD BANK ORDER

Materials Needed   Black ink pen

Red ink pen (depending on hospital policy)

Pencil

Eraser

Kardex form used in Activity 14–8

Patient ID labels

Blood bank requisition (if using requisition method)

Consent for transfusion(s) form

Computer and Practice Activity Software for Transcription of Physicians' Orders

Directions

Refer to Physicians' Order Sheet 14–9 in your patient's chart. Practice transcribing the blood bank order by following the steps below. Check with your instructor for variations of the procedure to adapt it to the practice in your area. Place a check mark (✓) in the box as you complete each step.

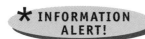
✱ INFORMATION ALERT!

Because receiving blood of the wrong type could cause the death of a patient, mislabeled specimens will be discarded and the patient will have to have the blood redrawn to be typed and crossmatched. The name on the computer screen and the patient ID label on the specimen should always be checked against the order with the doctors' order in the chart by the health unit coordinator before sending specimens to laboratory to avoid this situation.

Steps for Transcribing a Blood Bank Order

1. Read the order. ❑

2. Obtain the Kardex form and requisition form if using the requisition method and a consent for transfusion(s) form. ❑

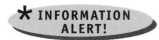
✱ INFORMATION ALERT!

A signed consent form for blood or a blood product transfusion is required. A patient may also sign a refusal form for blood or blood product transfusions. Refer to Chapter 8 in *Health Unit Coordinating*, 5th edition.

3. Order the blood component from the blood bank.

Use the computer method by:

a. labeling the blood transfusion consent form with patient ID label ❑

b. writing in the pertinent information on the consent form ❑

c. give the consent form to the patient's nurse to have patient sign ❑

d. selecting Enter Orders on the master screen ❑

e. selecting the patient's name from the census on the viewing screen ❑

f. selecting the laboratory department from the department menu on the viewing screen ❑

g. selecting the blood bank division from the laboratory department viewing screen ❑

h. typing in the pertinent information ❑

i. selecting the blood component to be ordered from the menu on the viewing screen and entering the crossmatch, if ordered ❑

j. entering the number of units to be ordered from the menu on the viewing screen ❑

k. writing "ord" or the computer order number in ink above each order on the doctors' order sheet to indicate that the blood has been ordered ❑

l. sending the order by pressing "enter" on the computer keyboard ❑

Use the requisition method by:

a. labeling the blood bank requisition and the consent form with patient ID label ❑

b. writing in the pertinent information on the consent form ❑

c. give the consent form to the patient's nurse to have patient sign ❑

d. writing in the pertinent information on the requisition ❑

e. placing a check mark (✓) in the box next to the blood component that has been ordered and a check mark (✓) in the box next to the crossmatch, if ordered ❑

f. writing the number of units in the appropriate space ❑

g. writing "ord" in ink above each order on the doctors' order sheet to indicate that the blood has been ordered ❑

h. sending the requisition ❑

4. Kardex the order by:

a. writing the date and the order in pencil in the lab column on the Kardex form ❑

b. writing the symbol "K" in ink in front of the order on the doctor's order sheet to indicate completion of the kardexing step ❑

5. Recheck each step for accuracy. ❑

6. Sign off the order to indicate completion of transcription. ❑

Place a check mark (✔) in the box below to indicate that you have completed Activity 14–9.

 Transcribe a Blood Bank Order   Date: _____

ACTIVITY 14-10

TRANSCRIBE URINALYSIS/URINE CHEMISTRY ORDERS

Materials Needed   Black ink pen

Red ink pen (depending on hospital policy)

Pencil

Eraser

Kardex form used in Activity 14–9

Patient ID labels (if using requisition method)

Laboratory requisitions (if using requisition method)

Computer and Practice Activity Software for Transcription of Physicans' Orders

Directions

Refer to Physicians' Order Sheet 14–10 in your patient's chart. Practice transcribing the urinalysis orders by following the steps below. Check with your instructor for variations of the procedure to adapt it to the practice in your area. Place a check mark (✓) in the box as you complete each step.

Steps for Transcribing Urinalysis/Urine Chemistry Orders

1. Read the orders. ❑

2. Obtain the Kardex form, requisition forms if using the requisition method, and labels. ❑

3. Order the test(s) from the laboratory department.

Use the computer method by:

a. selecting the patient's name from the census on the viewing screen ❑

b. selecting the laboratory department from the department menu on the viewing screen ❑

c. selecting the urinalysis/urine chemistry division from the laboratory department viewing screen ❑

d. selecting Enter Orders on the master screen ❑

e. typing in the pertinent information ❑

f. selecting the test(s) to be ordered from the menu on the viewing screen ❑

g. writing "ord" in ink above each order on the doctors' order sheet to indicate that the test has been ordered ❑

h. when collected, check label on specimen for proper patient ID, date, and time collected and for initials of person who collected specimen ❑

i. sending the specimen with copy of order ❑

> ✳ **INFORMATION ALERT!**
>
> Usually the order is entered into the computer when the specimen is obtained. The specimen is then sent to the laboratory with a copy of the information entered into the computer.

Use the requisition method by:

a. labeling the laboratory requisition with patient ID label ❑

> ✳ **INFORMATION ALERT!**
>
> Each urine specimen may require a separate requisition and label, as the specimens may go to different divisions of the laboratory (i.e., urine osmolality would be done in Chemistry and urine culture and sensitivity would be done in Microbiology).

b. writing in the pertinent information on the requisition ❑

c. placing a check mark (✓) in the column next to the test(s) to be ordered ❑

d. writing "ord" in ink above each order on the doctors' order sheet to indicate that the test has been ordered ❑

e. when collected, checking label on specimen for proper patient ID, date, and time collected and for initials of person who collected specimen ❑

f. sending specimen with requisition to the laboratory ❑

4. Kardex the orders by:

a. writing the date and the order in pencil in the lab column on the Kardex form ❑

b. writing the symbol "K" in ink in front of the order on the doctors' order sheet to indicate completion of the kardexing step ❑

5. Recheck each step for accuracy. ❑

6. Sign off the orders to indicate completion of transcription. ❑

Place a check mark (✔) in the box below to indicate that you have completed Activity 14–10.

❑ Transcribe Urinalysis/Urine Chemistry Orders   Date: _____

ACTIVITY 14-11

TRANSCRIBE CEREBROSPINAL FLUID ORDERS

Materials Needed
Black ink pen
Red ink pen (depending on hospital policy)
Pencil
Eraser
Kardex form used in Activity 14–10
Patient ID labels (if using requisition method)
Laboratory requisition (if using requisition method)
CSD requisition (if using requisition method)
Consent form
Computer and Practice Activity Software for Transcription of Physicians' Orders

Directions

Refer to Physicians' Order Sheet 14–11 in your patient's chart. Practice transcribing the cerebrospinal fluid orders by following the steps below. Check with your instructor for variations of the procedure to adapt it to the practice in your area. Place a check mark (✓) in the box as you complete each step.

Steps for Transcribing Cerebrospinal Fluid Orders

1. Read the orders. ❑

2. Obtain the Kardex form, requisition form if using the requisition method, consent form, and patient ID labels. ❑

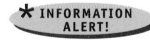

A lumbar puncture is an invasive procedure used to obtain cerebral spinal fluid. A consent form must be prepared and signed by the patient. Refer to Activity 8–3 for the steps to prepare a consent form. The consent order is usually transcribed onto the Kardex form. A spinal tap tray will need to be ordered if not on the CSD supply locker.

3. Order the test(s) from the laboratory department.

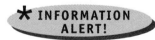

Specimens should be bagged and labeled with patient ID and the date, time, and initials of the person who collected the specimen. Indicate the tube number next to the test on the requisition. The numbers refer to the first specimen of fluid obtained (#1), the second specimen of fluid (#2), and the third specimen of fluid (#3). Numbers are etched on the specimen bottles. The doctor will indicate which test he or she wants on each tube by number.

Use the computer method by:

a. selecting Enter Orders on the master screen
b. selecting the patient's name from the census on the viewing screen ❑

c. selecting the laboratory department from the department menu on the viewing screen ☐

d. selecting thc body fluids division from the laboratory department viewing screen ☐

e. typing in the pertinent information ☐

f. selecting the body cavity source from the menu on the viewing screen ☐

g. selecting the tests to be ordered from the menu on the viewing screen ☐

h. writing "ord" in ink above each order on the doctors' order sheet to indicate that the test has been ordered ☐

i. check each label for proper patient ID, date, and time collected and for the initials of the person who collected the specimen ☐

j. sending the specimens with a copy of the order from the computer ☐

✴ INFORMATION ALERT!

Usually the order is entered into the computer when the specimen is obtained. Attach a copy of the order from the computer. Because this specimen is obtained by an invasive procedure, it cannot be sent by a tube system. It must be hand carried to the laboratory.

Use the requisition method by:

a. labeling the requisition with patient ID labels ☐

b. writing in the pertinent information ☐

c. placing a check mark (✓) in the column next to the test(s) to be ordered ☐

d. writing "ord" in ink above each order on the doctors' order sheet to indicate that the test has been ordered ☐

e. check each label for proper patient ID, date, and time collected and for the initials of the person who collected the specimen ☐

f. sending the specimens with the requisition ☐

4. Kardex the orders by:

a. writing the date and order in pencil in the lab column on the Kardex form ☐

b. writing the symbol "K" in ink in front of the order on the doctors' order sheet to indicate completion of the kardexing step ☐

5. Recheck each step for accuracy. ☐

6. Sign off the orders to indicate completion of transcription. ☐

Place a check mark (✓) in the box below to indicate that you have completed Activity 14–11.

☐ Transcribe Cerebrospinal Fluid Orders   Date: _____

ACTIVITY 14-12

TRANSCRIBE A REVIEW SET OF LABORATORY ORDERS

Materials Needed   Black ink pen

Red ink pen (depending on hospital policy)

Pencil

Eraser

Kardex form used in Activity 14–11

Patient ID labels (if using requisition method)

Laboratory requisitions (if using requisition method)

Computer and Practice Activity Software for Transcription of Physicians' Orders

Directions

Refer to Physicians' Order Sheet 14–12 in your patient's chart. Transcribe the orders. Refer to previous laboratory activities for the appropriate transcription steps as needed.

Steps for Transcribing a Review Set of Laboratory Orders

1. Read the orders. ❑

2. Check orders for stats. ❑

3. Obtain the Kardex form, requisition forms if using the requisition method, and labels. ❑

4. Order as necessary. ❑

5. Kardex the orders. ❑

6. Recheck each step for accuracy. ❑

7. Sign off the orders to indicate completion of transcription. ❑

Place a check mark (✔) in the box below to indicate that you have completed Activity 14–12.

❑ Transcribe a Review Set of Laboratory Orders   Date: _____

ACTIVITY 14-13

TRANSCRIBE A REVIEW SET OF DOCTORS' ORDERS

Materials Needed

Black ink pen

Red ink pen (depending on hospital policy)

Pencil

Yellow highlighter

Eraser

Kardex form and MAR used in previous chapters

Patient ID labels (if using requisition method)

Necessary requisitions and forms

Directions

Refer to Physicians' Order Sheet 14–13 in your patient's chart. Transcribe the orders. Refer to the previous activities for the appropriate transcription steps as needed.

Steps for Transcribing a Review Set of Doctors' Orders

1. Read the complete set of doctors' orders. ❑

2. Send pharmacy copy. ❑

3. Check orders for stats. ❑

4. Make any necessary phone calls. ❑

5. Obtain all necessary forms. ❑

6. Order as necessary. ❑

7. Kardex the orders. ❑

8. Record medications on the MAR. ❑

9. Recheck each step for accuracy. ❑

10. Sign off the orders to indicate completion of transcription. ❑

Suggestion to the student: Use this space to list the forms you will need.

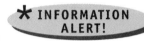

✱ INFORMATION ALERT!

Transcribing doctors' orders is a critical task, and an error could cause harm to a patient. If you are not absolutely sure in interpreting the doctors' orders, ask the patient's nurse or the doctor who wrote the orders.

Place a check mark (✔) in the box below to indicate that you have completed Activity 14–13.

☐ Transcribe a Review Set of Doctors' Orders   Date: _____

ACTIVITY 14-14

RECORD TELEPHONED DOCTORS' ORDERS

Materials Needed   Pen
                            Physicians' order sheet

Directions

Practice recording the telephoned physicians' orders printed below by following the steps below. Place a check mark (✔) in the box as you complete each step.

Telephoned Physicians' Orders

"This is Dr. Paul Pinrod with some orders on Mary Copa. Ready?

Stat complete blood cell count and electrolytes

Comprehensive chem panel at 0600

Total iron-binding capacity in the morning

Type and crossmatch two units of packed cells to be transfused when ready.

I will be there in about an hour to do a lumbar puncture; please have the tray, size eight and one-half gloves, and a bottle of liquid iodine at the bedside.

Have the consent signed.

I will want a cell count and differential on tube number 1, protein and glucose on tube number 2, and culture and sensitivity on tube number 3.

Read those back to me please.

Thank you."

Steps for Recording Telephoned Physicians' Orders

1. Have someone read the above orders to you while you record them on a physicians' order form. ❑
2. Use accepted abbreviations and symbols as you write the orders. ❑
3. For further practice, obtain a new Kardex and practice transcribing the orders you have written. ❑

Place a check mark (✔) in the box below to indicate that you have completed Activity 14–14.

❑ Record Telephoned Doctors' Orders   Date: _____

ACTIVITY 14-15

RECORD TELEPHONE MESSAGES

Materials Needed   Pen or pencil
                         Message pad

Directions

Practice recording the telephone messages printed below by following the steps below. Place a check mark (✔) in the box as you complete each step.

Telephone Messages

1. "Hi, This is Pat in chemistry. Would you check with Dr. Black to find out if the potassium that she ordered on Johnny Smith this afternoon can be run on the blood we have on him from this morning?" ❑

2. "This is John in urinalysis. Please let Susan Garcias' nurse know that there is insufficient quantity to do a complete urinalysis on the specimen that she sent us." ❑

Steps for Recording Telephone Messages

1. Have someone read the above messages to you while you record them on a message pad. ❑
2. Write down who the message is for. ❑
3. Write down the caller's name. ❑
4. Write down the date and time of the call. ❑
5. Write down the purpose of the call. ❑
6. If a return call is expected, write down the number to call. ❑
7. Sign your name to the message. ❑

Place a check mark (✔) in the box below to indicate that you have completed Activity 14–15.

❑ Record Telephone Messages   Date: _____

ACTIVITY 14-16

RECORD TELEPHONED LABORATORY RESULTS

Materials Needed   Pen or pencil
                        Lab result form

Directions

Practice recording the laboratory results printed below by following the steps below. Place a check mark (✔) in the box as you complete each step.

Telephoned Laboratory Results

1. "Hi, this is Jeannie from chemistry in the lab. I have stat electrolyte results on Terita Banks. Are you ready?

Sodium = 136 mEq/L

Potassium = 3.8 mEq/L

Chloride = 106 mEq/L

CO_2 = 21 mEq/L

Please repeat those back to me. Thanks."

2. "This is Chuck from hematology in the lab. I have PT and PTT results on Frances Key.

PT was 12.0 seconds

PTT was 24.2 seconds

Repeat those please. Thanks."

3. "This is Jennifer from chemistry in the lab with a critical potassium value on Megan Morgan. The potassium was 7.2—this was a finger stick. Please repeat the value and ask the resident if she would like a repeat venous specimen drawn and run. May I have your name again please? Thanks."

4. "Hi, this is Joe from chemistry in the lab. I have stat cardiac enzymes on Pat Tagler. Ready?

CPK = 250 mU/mL

LDH = 200 mU/mL

SGOT = 45 u/mL

Would you repeat those results please? Thanks."

Steps for Recording Telephoned Laboratory Results

1. Have someone read the above results to you while you record them on a laboratory result form.   ❑

2. Repeat the results back to the person giving them to you.   ❑

3. Record the name of the person giving you the results. ❑

4. Notify the patient's nurse of the results and, if necessary (requested to do so by the nurse or previously requested to do so by resident or doctor), the patient's resident or doctor. ❑

Place a check mark (✔) in the box below to indicate that you have completed Activity 14–16.

❑ Record Telephone Laboratory Results   Date: _____

PHYSICIANS' ORDER SHEET 14–1

DATE	TIME	SYMBOL	ORDERS
			CBC ⎫
			LE cell prep ⎬ today
			Eosinophil smear ⎭
			Dr

PHYSICIANS' ORDER SHEET 14–2

DATE	TIME	SYMBOL	ORDERS
			Daily H & H ⎫ starting
			PT qd ⎬ in AM
			Dr

PHYSICIANS' ORDER SHEET 14–3

DATE	TIME	SYMBOL	ORDERS
			BUN ⎫
			Lytes ⎬ this AM
			Acid phos ⎬
			Uric acid ⎭
			Dr

PHYSICIANS' ORDER SHEET 14–4

DATE	TIME	SYMBOL	ORDERS
			STAT LDH, AST & CK
			RBS now
			Dr

PHYSICIANS' ORDER SHEET 14–5

DATE	TIME	SYMBOL	ORDERS
			FBS
			Cholesterol ⎫ in AM
			Triglycerides
			Fe, TIBC
			Dr

PHYSICIANS' ORDER SHEET 14–6

DATE	TIME	SYMBOL	ORDERS
			D/C daily H & H & PT
			STAT lytes
			2 hr PPBS today
			Serum osmolality today
			Daily FBS
			TSH in AM
			Vancomycin peak & trough around 3rd dose
			Dr

PHYSICIANS' ORDER SHEET 14–7

DATE	TIME	SYMBOL	ORDERS
			Reflex Ua
			Sputum for AFB culture
			Sputum for C & S
			Stool x 3 for O & P
			Dr

PHYSICIANS' ORDER SHEET 14–8

DATE	TIME	SYMBOL	ORDERS
			RA factor ⎫
			Monospot ⎬ today
			HbsAg ⎭
			Dr

PHYSICIANS' ORDER SHEET 14–9

DATE	TIME	SYMBOL	ORDERS
			T & X-match 2 units PC for transfusion today
			Dr

PHYSICIANS' ORDER SHEET 14–10

DATE	TIME	SYMBOL	ORDERS
			Route Ua
			Urine osmolality
			Dr

PHYSICIANS' ORDER SHEET 14–11

DATE	TIME	SYMBOL	ORDERS
			Have consent signed for LP per Dr Jack Rabbit
			CSF to lab for:
			tube #1 cell ct c̄ diff
			#2 protein & glucose
			#3 C & S
			Dr

PHYSICIANS' ORDER SHEET 14–12

DATE	TIME	SYMBOL	ORDERS
			ESR & creatinine
			CKMP panel & troponin
			Bilirubin total today
			Cocci screen
			CMP in AM
			Dr

PHYSICIANS' ORDER SHEET 14–13

DATE	TIME	SYMBOL	ORDERS
			△ diet to 1500 cal ADA-NSA
			BRP c̄ help
			Obtain ETS
			D/C foley—may st cath x 1 if unable to void p̄ 8 hr
			Convert IV to heplock c̄ rout saline flushes
			D/C PICC
			D/C Atenolol
			D/C HCTZ
			Claraseptic throat spray q 3 hr prn for throat irritation
			Maalox 30 cc q 3-4 hr prn for upset stomach
			Lopressor 50 mg po qd
			C & S rt ear drainage
			Lanoxin peak level 2° p̄ 5pm dose
			Dr

Diagnostic Imaging Orders

Place the Physicians' Order Sheets located at the end of the chapter in your patient's chart. Follow the directions for each activity to transcribe orders.

Activities in This Chapter

 ## ACTIVITY 15-1

TRANSCRIBE RADIOLOGY ORDERS THAT DO NOT REQUIRE PREPARATION OR CONTRAST MEDIUM

Materials Needed

Black ink pen

Red ink pen (depending on hospital policy)

Pencil

Eraser

Kardex form used in previous chapters

Patient ID labels (if using requisition method)

Diagnostic imaging requisition (if using requisition method)

Computer and Practice Activity Software for Transcription of Physicians' Orders

Directions

Refer to Physicians' Order Sheet 15–1 in your patient's chart. Practice transcribing the radiology orders by following the steps below. Check with your instructor for variations of the procedure to adapt it to the practice in your area. Place a check mark (✓) in the box as you complete each step.

Steps for Transcribing Radiology (X-ray Orders That Do Not Require Preparation or Contrast Medium)

1. Read the orders. ❑

2. Obtain the Kardex form and requisition if using the requisition method. ❑

3. Order the study (studies) from the diagnostic imaging department.

Use the computer method by:
a. selecting Enter Orders on the master screen ❑
b. selecting the patient's name from the census on the viewing screen ❑
c. selecting the diagnostic imaging department from the department menu on the viewing screen
d. selecting the appropriate division from the diagnostic imaging divisions screen
e. typing in the pertinent data; answering all questions asked on computer screen (i.e., reason for examination, transportation method, is patient on oxygen, does patient have an IV) ❑
f. entering the study (studies) to be performed ❑
g. entering the date the study (studies) is (are) to be performed under the appropriate heading ❑
h. writing "ord" in ink above each order on the doctors' order sheet to indicate that the study has been ordered ❑
i. sending the order by pressing "enter" on the computer keyboard ❑

Use the requisition method by:
a. labeling the diagnostic imaging requisition with patient ID label ❑
b. writing in the pertinent information; answering all questions asked on requisition (i.e., reason for examination, transportation method, is patient on oxygen, does patient have an IV) ❑
c. writing the order under the heading "Examination Requested" ❑
d. writing the date the study (studies) is (are) to be performed in the appropriate space ❑
e. writing "ord" in ink above each order on the doctors' order sheet to indicate that the study has been ordered ❑
f. sending the requisition ❑

4. Kardex the orders by:
a. writing the date and order in pencil in the diagnostic imaging column on the Kardex form ❑
b. writing in pencil the date the radiology study will be performed in the column next to the order ❑
c. writing the symbol "K" in ink in front of the order on the doctors' order sheet to indicate completion of the kardexing step ❑

5. Recheck each step for accuracy. ❑

6. Sign off the orders to indicate completion of transcription. ❑

Place a check mark (✔) in the box below to indicate that you have completed Activity 15–1.

❑ Transcribe Radiology Orders That Do Not Require Preparation or Contrast Medium   Date: _____

ACTIVITY 15-2

TRANSCRIBE RADIOLOGY ORDERS THAT REQUIRE PREPARATION AND CONTRAST MEDIUM

Materials Needed: Black ink pen
Red ink pen (depending on hospital policy)
Pencil
Eraser
Kardex form used in Activity 15–1
Labeled MAR used in previous chapters
Patient ID labels (if using requisition method)
Diet requisition (if using requisition method)
Diagnostic requisitions (if using requisition method)
Diagnostic imaging routine preparation cards (printed at end of this chapter)
Computer and Practice Activity Software for Transcription of Physicians' Orders

Directions

Refer to Physicians' Order Sheet 15–2 in your patient's chart. Practice transcribing the radiology orders by following the steps below. Check with your instructor for variations of the procedure in your area. Place a check mark (✓) in the box as you complete each step.

Steps for Transcribing Radiology Orders That Do Require Preparation and Contrast Medium

1. Read the orders. ☐

2. Obtain the Kardex form; requisitions, if using the requisition method; or prep cards; and MAR. ☐

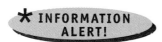
✱ INFORMATION ALERT!

Many health care facility computer systems will automatically provide a printout of the appropriate diagnostic imaging preparation when the examination is ordered.

3. Order the study (studies) from the diagnostic imaging department.

Use the computer method by:
a. selecting Enter Orders on the master screen ☐
b. selecting the patient's name from the census on the viewing screen ☐
c. selecting the diagnostic imaging department from the department menu on the viewing screen ☐
d. selecting the appropriate division from the diagnostic imaging divisions screen ☐
e. typing in the pertinent data; answering all questions asked on the computer screen (i.e., reason for examination, transportation method, is patient on oxygen, does patient have an IV) ☐
f. entering the study (studies) to be performed ☐
g. entering the date the study (studies) is (are) to be performed under the appropriate heading ☐
h. writing "ord" in ink above each order on the doctors' order sheet to indicate that the study has been ordered ☐
i. sending the order by pressing "enter" on the computer keyboard ☐
j. placing the diagnostic imaging preparation printout in the patient's Kardex ☐

Use the requisition method by:

a. labeling the diagnostic imaging requisition with patient ID label ❑

b. writing in the pertinent information; answering all questions asked on requisition (i.e., reason for examination, transportation method, is patient on oxygen, does patient have an IV) ❑

c. writing the order under the heading "Examination Requested" ❑

d. writing the date the study (studies) is (are) to be performed in the appropriate space ❑

e. writing "ord" in ink above each order on the doctors' order sheet to indicate that the study has been ordered ❑

f. Sending the requisition ❑

g. Placing the diagnostic imaging preparation card in the patient's Kardex ❑

4. Order the diet change from the dietary department by entering the diet change into the computer or by using the diet requisition form (refer to the dietary activities in Chapter 12 in this manual). ❑

5. Kardex the orders by:

a. writing the date and order in pencil in the diagnostic imaging column on the Kardex form ❑

b. writing in pencil the date the radiology study will be performed in the column next to the order ❑

c. writing the symbol "K" in ink in front of the order on the doctors' order sheet to indicate completion of the kardexing step ❑

★ INFORMATION ALERT!

The preparation computer printout or card is often placed with the patient's Kardex form in the Kardex; therefore, the preparation and diet for the procedure may not be written on the Kardex form.

6. Record the preparation medication in ink on the MAR under the correct heading by:

a. writing (1) today's date; (2) the name of the medication; (3) the dosage; (4) the route of administration; (5) the time of administration; and (6) the date of administration ❑

b. writing the symbol "m" in ink in front of the order on the doctors' order sheet to indicate completion of this step of transcription ❑

7. Recheck each step for accuracy. ❑

8. Sign off the orders to indicate completion of transcription. ❑

Place a check mark (✔) in the box below to indicate that you have completed Activity 15–2.

❑ Transcribe Radiology Orders That Require Preparation and Contrast Medium

Date: _____

ACTIVITY 15-3

TRANSCRIBE A SPECIAL RADIOLOGY PROCEDURE ORDER

Materials Needed:

Black ink pen

Red ink pen (depending on hospital policy)

Pencil

Eraser

Kardex form used in Activity 15–2

Labeled MAR used in Activity 15–2

Patient ID labels

Diet requisition (if using requisition method)

Diagnostic imaging requisition (if using requisition method)

Consent to operation, administration of anesthetics, and the rendering of other medical services form

Computer and Practice Activity Software for Transcription of Physicians' Orders

Directions

Refer to Physicians' Order Sheet 15–3 in your patient's chart. Practice transcribing the special radiology procedure order and related orders by following the steps below. Check with your instructor for variations of the procedure to adapt it to the practice in your area. Place a check mark (✓) in the box as you complete each step.

Steps for Transcribing a Special Radiology Procedure Order

1. Read the order. ❑

2. Obtain the Kardex form and requisition form if using the requisition method, MAR, and consent form. ❑

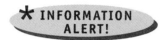
✱ INFORMATION ALERT!

A myelogram is an invasive procedure. A consent form must be prepared and signed by the patient.

Refer to Activity 8–2 for the steps to prepare a consent form. The consent form is usually transcribed into the Kardex form.

3. Order the procedure from the diagnostic imaging department.

Use the computer method by:
a. labeling and writing in the procedure on the consent form ❑
b. giving the consent form to the patient's nurse to have patient sign ❑
c. selecting Enter Orders on the master screen ❑
d. selecting the patient's name from the census on the viewing screen ❑
e. selecting the diagnostic imaging department from the department menu on the viewing screen ❑
f. selecting the appropriate division from the diagnostic imaging divisions screen ❑
g. typing in the pertinent data; answering all questions asked on the computer screen (i.e., reason for examination, transportation method, is patient on oxygen, does patient have an IV) ❑
h. entering the procedure to be performed ❑
i. entering the date the procedure is to be performed under the appropriate heading ❑
j. writing "ord" in ink above each order on the doctors' order sheet to indicate that the procedure has been ordered ❑
k. sending the order by pressing "enter" on the computer keyboard ❑

Use the requisition method by:
a. labeling and writing in the procedure on the consent form ❑
b. giving the consent form to the patient's nurse to have patient sign ❑
c. labeling the diagnostic imaging requisition with patient ID label ❑
d. writing in the pertinent information; answering all questions asked on the requisition (i.e., reason for examination, transportation method, is patient on oxygen, does patient have an IV) ❑
e. writing the order under the heading "Examination Requested" ❑
f. writing the date the procedure is to be performed in the appropriate space ❑
g. writing "ord" in ink above each order on the doctors' order sheet to indicate that the procedure has been ordered ❑
h. sending the requisition ❑

4. Order the diet change from the dietary department by using the computer method or the requisition method (refer to the dietary activities in Chapter 12 in this manual). ❑

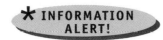

✱ INFORMATION ALERT!

The patient is usually kept NPO for special procedures.

5. Kardex the radiology order by:
   a. writing the date and order in pencil in the diagnostic imaging column on the Kardex form ❑
   b. writing in pencil the date the radiology procedure will be done in the column next to the order ❑
   c. writing the symbol "K" in ink in front of the order on the doctors' order sheet to indicate that the order has been kardexed ❑

6. Kardex the diet change by:
   a. writing the date and order in pencil in the diet column on the Kardex form ❑
   b. writing the symbol "K" in ink in front of the order on the doctors' order sheet to indicate that the diet change has been kardexed ❑

7. Record the medications in ink on the MAR under the correct heading by:
   a. writing (1) today's date; (2) the name of the medication; (3) the dosage; (4) the route of administration; (5) the time of administration; and (6) the date of administration ❑
   b. writing the symbol "m" in ink in front of the order on the doctors' order sheet to indicate completion of this step of transcription ❑

8. Recheck each step for accuracy. ❑

9. Sign off the orders to indicate completion of transcription. ❑

Place a check mark (✔) in the box below to indicate that you have completed Activity 15–3.

❑ Transcribe a Special Radiology Procedure Order   Date: _____

ACTIVITY 15-4

TRANSCRIBE A COMPUTED TOMOGRAPHY ORDER, AN ULTRASOUND ORDER, AND A MAGNETIC RESONANCE IMAGING ORDER

Materials Needed   Black ink pen
                         Red ink pen (depending on hospital policy)
                         Pencil
                         Eraser
                         Kardex form used in Activity 15–3
                         Computer and Practice Activity Software for Transcription of Physicians' Orders

Directions

Refer to Physicians' Order Sheet 15–4 in your patient's chart. Practice transcribing the diagnostic imaging orders by following the steps below. Check with your instructor for variations of the procedure to adapt it to the practice in your area. Place a check mark (✔) in the box as you complete each step.

Steps for Transcribing a Computed Tomography Order, an Ultrasound Order, and a Magnetic Resonance Imaging Order

1. Read the orders. ❑

2. Obtain the Kardex form and requisition forms if using the requisition method. ❑

3. Order the study (studies) from the diagnostic imaging department. ❑

Use the computer method by:
a. selecting Enter Orders on the master screen ❑
b. selecting the patient's name from the census on the viewing screen ❑
c. selecting the diagnostic imaging department from the department menu on the viewing screen ❑
d. selecting the appropriate division from the diagnostic imaging divisions screen ❑
e. typing in the pertinent data; answering all questions on the computer screen (i.e., reason for examination, transportation method, is patient on oxygen, does patient have an IV) ❑
f. entering the study to be performed ❑
g. entering the date the study is to be performed under the appropriate heading ❑
h. writing "ord" in ink above each order on the doctors' order sheet to indicate that the study has been ordered ❑
i. sending the order by pressing "enter" on the computer keyboard ❑

Use the requisition method by:
a. labeling the diagnostic imaging requisitions with patient ID labels ❑
b. writing in the pertinent information; answering all questions asked on the requisition (i.e., reason for examination, transportation method, is patient on oxygen, does patient have an IV) ❑
c. writing the order under the heading "Examination Requested" ❑
d. writing the date the study is to be performed in the appropriate space ❑
e. writing "ord" in ink above each order on the doctors' order sheet to indicate that the study has been ordered ❑

> ✱ **INFORMATION ALERT!**
>
> The patient may be kept NPO for some CT, US, or MRI procedures. Check with your instructor for direction.

4. Order the diet change if necessary from the dietary department by using the computer method or the requisition method (refer to the dietary activities in Chapter 12 in this manual). ❑

> ✱ **INFORMATION ALERT!**
>
> The studies may need to be entered separately into the computer, or separate requisitions used as each may be performed by a different division in the diagnostic imaging department.

5. Kardex the orders by:
a. writing the date and order in pencil in the diagnostic imaging column on the Kardex form ❑
b. writing in pencil the date the radiology study will be performed in the column next to the order ❑
c. writing the symbol "K" in ink in front of the order on the doctors' order sheet to indicate completion of the kardexing step ❑

6. Recheck each step for accuracy. ❑

7. Sign off the orders to indicate completion of transcription. ❑

Place a check mark (✔) in the box below to indicate that you have completed Activity 15–4.

☐ Transcribe a Computed Tomography Order, an Ultrasound Order, and a Magnetic Resonance Imaging Order

Date: _____

ACTIVITY 15-5

TRANSCRIBE A NUCLEAR MEDICINE ORDER

Materials Needed　　Black ink pen
Red ink pen (depending on hospital policy)
Pencil
Eraser
Kardex form used in Activity 15–4
Patient ID labels (if using requisition method)
Diagnostic imaging requisition (if using requisition method)
Computer and Practice Activity Software for Transcription of Physicians' Orders

Directions

Refer to Physicians' Order Sheet 15–5 in your patient's chart. Practice transcribing the nuclear medicine order by following the steps below. Check with your instructor for variations of the procedure to adapt it to the practice in your area. Place a check mark (✔) in the box as you complete each step.

Steps for Transcribing a Nuclear Medicine Order

1. Read the order.　　　　　　　　　　　　　　　　　　　　　　　　　　　　　☐

2. Obtain the Kardex form.

3. Order the study from the diagnostic imaging department.

Use the computer method by:
a. selecting Enter Orders on the master screen　　　　　　　　　　　　　　　☐
b. selecting the patient's name from the census on the viewing screen　　　　☐
c. selecting the diagnostic imaging department from the department menu on the
viewing screen　　　　　　　　　　　　　　　　　　　　　　　　　　　　☐
d. selecting the nuclear medicine division from the viewing screen　　　　　☐
e. typing in the pertinent data; answering all questions on the requisition (i.e., reason
for examination, transportation method, is patient on oxygen, does patient have an IV)　☐
f. entering the study to be performed　　　　　　　　　　　　　　　　　　　☐
g. entering the date the study is to be performed under the appropriate heading　☐
h. writing "ord" in ink above each order on the doctors'
order sheet to indicate that the study has been ordered　　　　　　　　　☐
i. sending the order by pressing "enter" on the computer keyboard　　　　　☐

Use the requisition method by:
a. obtaining and labeling the diagnostic imaging requisition with patient ID label　☐
b. writing in the pertinent information; answering all questions on the requisition (i.e., reason
for examination, transportation method, is patient on oxygen, does patient have an IV)　☐
c. writing the order under the heading "Examination Requested"　　　　　　☐
d. writing the date the study is to be performed in the appropriate space　　　☐
e. writing "ord" in ink above each order on the doctors' order sheet to indicate that
the study has been ordered　　　　　　　　　　　　　　　　　　　　　　☐
f. sending the requisition

4. Kardex the orders by:
   a. writing the date and order in pencil in the diagnostic imaging column on the Kardex form ❑
   b. writing in pencil the date the radiology study will be performed in the column next to the order ❑
   c. writing the symbol "K" in ink in front of the order on the doctors' order sheet to indicate completion of the kardexing step ❑
5. Recheck each step for accuracy. ❑
6. Sign off the orders to indicate completion of transcription. ❑

Place a check mark (✔) in the box below to indicate that you have completed Activity 15–5.

❑ Transcribe a Nuclear Medicine Order   Date: _____

ACTIVITY 15-6

TRANSCRIBE A REVIEW SET OF DOCTORS' ORDERS

Materials Needed
Black ink pen
Red ink pen (depending on hospital policy)
Pencil
Eraser
Yellow highlighter
Kardex form used in Activity 15–5
Patient ID labels
Necessary requisitions and forms
Computer and Practice Activity Software for Transcription of Physicians' Orders

Directions

Refer to Physicians' Order Sheet 15–6 in your patient's chart. Transcribe the orders. Refer to the previous activities for the appropriate transcription steps as needed.

Steps for Transcribing a Review Set of Doctors' Orders

1. Read the orders. ❑
2. Send or fax pharmacy copy. ❑
3. Check orders for stats. ❑
4. Make any necessary phone calls. ❑
5. Obtain all necessary forms and radiology preparation cards. ❑
6. Order as necessary. ❑
7. Kardex the order. ❑
8. Record medications on the MAR. ❑
9. Recheck each step for accuracy. ❑
10. Sign off the orders to indicate completion of transcription. ❑

Suggestion to the student: Use this space to list the forms you will need.

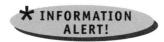 **INFORMATION ALERT!**

Transcribing doctors' orders is a critical task, and an error could cause harm to a patient. If you are not absolutely sure in interpreting the doctors' orders, ask the patient's nurse or the doctor who wrote the orders.

Place a check mark (✓) in the box below to indicate that you have completed Activity 15–6.

☐ Transcribe a Review Set of Doctors' Orders   Date: _____

 ACTIVITY 15-7

RECORD TELEPHONED DOCTORS' ORDERS

Materials Needed   Pen
                              Physicians' order sheet

Directions

Practice recording the telephoned physicians' orders printed below by following the steps below. Place a check mark (✓) in the box as you complete each step.

Telephoned Physician's Orders

"Hello, this is Dr. Bones with orders on John Fracture. Ready?

Get a stat posteroanterior and lateral chest—for infiltrates

Computed tomography of brain—possible brain tumor

Ask Dr. Janet Picture to interpret the films and call me with her findings. Ask Mr. Fracture's family to meet me at the hospital this afternoon at 2 PM. Thank you."

Steps for Recording Telephoned Doctors' Orders

1. Have someone read the above orders to you while you record them on a physicians' order sheet. ❏

2. Use accepted abbreviations and symbols as you write the orders. ❏

3. For further practice, obtain a new Kardex and practice transcribing the orders you have written. ❏

Place a check mark (✔) in the box below to indicate that you have completed Activity 15–7.

❏ Record Telephoned Doctors' Orders   Date: _____

ACTIVITY 15-8

RECORDING TELEPHONE MESSAGES

Materials Needed   Pen or pencil

Message pad

Directions

Practice recording the telephone messages printed below by following the steps below. Place a check mark (✔) in the box as you complete each step.

Telephone Messages

1. "This is Paul in diagnostic imaging. We are ready for John Fracture to do his chest x-ray. Please notify his nurse that someone will be up in 5 minutes to pick him up."

2. "Hi, this is Cindy in computed tomography. Could you have John Fracture's nurse arrange to have him down for his computed tomography of the brain at one o'clock sharp? If there is a problem, please call me right back. Thanks."

3. "This is Paula in special procedures. Please ask Mary Copa's nurse to give the on-call medication ordered and we will be up to get her in one half hour. Thanks."

Steps for Recording Telephone Messages

1. Have someone read the above messages to you while you record them on a message pad ❏

2. Write down who the message is for. ❏

3. Write down the caller's name. ❏

4. Write down the date and time of the call. ❏

5. Write down the purpose of the call. ❏

6. If a return call is expected, write down the number to call. ❏

7. Sign your name to the message. ❏

Place a check mark (✔) in the box below to indicate that you have completed Activity 15–8.

❏ Record Telephone Messages   Date: _____

DIAGNOSTIC IMAGING ROUTINE PREPARATION CARDS

Directions

Cut appropriate preparation card along dotted line. Record medications (including packaged enemas) on your patient's medication record. Place the prep card in your patient's Kardex. Preparations for diagnostic procedures vary among hospitals. (Check with your instructor for any variations in these directions.)

IVU or IVP

Fleet enema this evening prior to test and in AM before procedure

Low-residue diet evening meal day before procedure

NPO 8–12 hours before procedure

Limit fluids to 600 cc PO for 18 hours before procedure

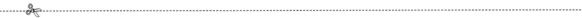

GB Series

Oral contrast medium PM before procedure

Light fat-free meal PM before procedure

NPO 8–12 hours before procedure

UGI–SBFT

NPO 8–12 hours before procedure

No smoking or gum chewing 8–12 hours before procedure

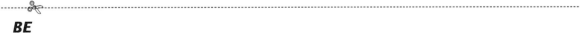

BE

Day before procedure:

2:00 PM: x-prep 1 bottle

7:00 PM: Dulcolax 2 tabs

NPO 2400 hrs

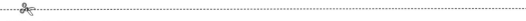

US of Abdomen

NPO 8–12 hours before procedure

Full bladder, drink fluids—Do not void

No smoking AM of exam

US of Pelvis

Full bladder, drink fluids—Do not void
May require H_2O enema

US of GB

Fat-free PM meal day before procedure
Fast 8–10 hours before test
No smoking AM of exam

PHYSICIANS' ORDER SHEET 15–1

DATE	TIME	SYMBOL	ORDERS
			PA & lat chest Cl: √ for infiltrates
			KUB Cl: poss obstruction
			Dr
			Mammogram Cl: tumor
			Dr

PHYSICIANS' ORDER SHEET 15–2

DATE	TIME	SYMBOL	ORDERS
			IVU Cl: poss ureterolithiasis
			BE Cl: √ for tumor
			Dr

PHYSICIANS' ORDER SHEET 15–3

DATE	TIME	SYMBOL	ORDERS
			Cervical myelogram @ 0830 in AM CI: ruptured disc
			Have consent signed
			Demerol 100 mg ⎤
			Phenegan 25 mg ⎦ IM @ 0730
			NPO 2400 hr
			Dr

PHYSICIANS' ORDER SHEET 15–4

DATE	TIME	SYMBOL	ORDERS
			CT scan of head DSA CI: poss aneurysm
			US of abd CI: abscess
			MRI of lt shoulder CI: torn rotator cuff
			Dr

PHYSICIANS' ORDER SHEET 15–5

DATE	TIME	SYMBOL	ORDERS
			Bone scan CI: poss metastasis
			Dr

PHYSICIANS' ORDER SHEET 15–6

DATE	TIME	SYMBOL	ORDERS
			△ diet to cl liq
			BR c̄ HOB ↑30°
			NVS q 2° x 3
			st cath for C & S
			Start IV of 1000 cc Isolyte M 120 cc/hr
			Use #18 needle—if IV infiltrates, call hospitalist
			p̄ urine obtained, start Cipro 250 mg po bid & Tylenol
			650 mg po q 4 hr prn
			D/C Lanoxin
			Transderm nitro 5 cm 2/2.5 mg to skin q 24 hr
			UGI c̄ SBFT Cl: peptic ulcer
			Lymphangiogram lt leg Cl: poss lymphatic obstruction
			X-ray rt tibia Cl: poss FX
			STAT CBC & plt ct
			6 U plts to be transfused today
			Dr

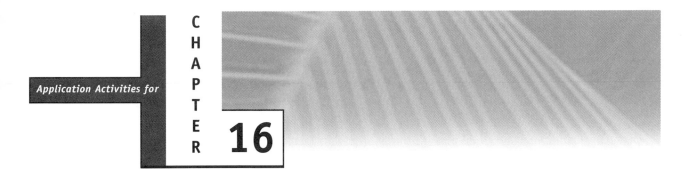

Other Diagnostic Studies

Place the Physicians' Order Sheets located at the end of the chapter in your patient's chart. Follow the directions for each activity to transcribe orders.

Activities in This Chapter

Transcribe
16–1: Cardiovascular Diagnostic Orders
16–2: Neurodiagnostics Order
16–3: Endoscopy Order
16–4: Respiratory Diagnostic Orders
16–5: A Review Set of Doctors' Orders

Record:
16–6: Telephoned Doctors' Orders
16–7: Telephone Messages

ACTIVITY 16-1

TRANSCRIBE CARDIOVASCULAR DIAGNOSTICS ORDERS

Materials Needed
Black ink pen
Red ink pen (depending on hospital policy)
Pencil
Eraser
Kardex form used in previous chapters
MAR used in previous chapters
Patient ID labels (if using the requisition method)
Cardiovascular diagnostics requisition (if using the requisition method)
Computer and Practice Activity Software for Transcription of Physicians' Orders

Directions

Refer to Physicians' Order Sheet 16–1 in your patient's chart. Practice transcribing the cardiovascular diagnostics orders by following the steps below. Check with your instructor for variations of the procedure to adapt it to the practice in your area. Place a check mark (✓) in the box as you complete each step.

Steps for Transcribing Cardiovascular Diagnostics Orders

1. Read the orders. ❑

2. Obtain the Kardex form and requisitions if using the requisition method. ❑

3. Order the study (studies) from the cardiovascular diagnostics department. It is important for the cardiologist interpreting the results of the study to know if the patient is taking cardiovascular medications. Refer to Chapter 13 in *Health Unit Coordinating*, 5th edition, for a list of cardiovascular medications. Record those that have been ordered for the patient on the requisition or enter the medications into the computer. ❑

Use the computer method by:
a. selecting Enter Orders on the master screen ❑
b. selecting the patient's name from the census on the viewing screen ❑
c. selecting the cardiovascular diagnostics department from the department menu on the viewing screen ❑
d. typing in the pertinent information (refer to your patient's MAR)—enter any cardiovascular medications onto the order screen ❑
e. entering the study to be performed ❑
f. entering the date the study is to be performed under the appropriate heading ❑
g. writing "ord" in ink above each order on the doctors' order sheet to indicate that the study has been ordered ❑
h. sending the order by pressing "enter" on the computer keyboard ❑

Use the requisition method by:
a. labeling the cardiovascular requisition with patient ID label ❑
b. writing in the pertinent information (refer to your patient's MAR)—write any cardiovascular medications that your patient is taking on the requisition ❑
c. placing a check mark (✓) in the box next to the study to be ordered ❑
d. writing the date and the study to be performed in the appropriate space ❑
e. writing "ord" in ink above each order on the doctors' order sheet to indicate that the study has been ordered ❑
f. sending the requisition ❑

✱ INFORMATION ALERT!

It is important to note any cardiovascular medications on the order for cardiovascular tests. Studies ordered on different days usually require ordering separately. Most health care facility computer systems have the function to order tests for future dates.

4. Kardex the orders by:
a. writing the date and order in pencil in the diagnostic studies column on the Kardex form ❑
b. writing in pencil the date that the cardiovascular study will be done in the column next to the order ❑
c. writing the symbol "K" in ink in front of the order on the doctors' order sheet to indicate completion of the kardexing step ❑

5. Recheck each step for accuracy. ❑

6. Sign off the orders to indicate completion of transcription. ❑

Place a check mark (✓) in the box below to indicate that you have completed Activity 16–1.

❑ Transcribe Cardiovascular Diagnostic Orders   Date: _____

ACTIVITY 16-2

TRANSCRIBE NEURODIAGNOSTIC ORDERS

Materials Needed   Black ink pen
Red ink pen (depending on hospital policy)
Pencil
Eraser
Kardex form used in Activity 16–1
MAR used in previous chapters
Patient ID labels
Neurodiagnostic requisition
Computer and Practice Activity Software for Transcription of Physicians' Orders

Directions

Refer to Physicians' Order Sheet 16–2 in your patient's chart. Practice transcribing the neurodiagnostics order following the steps below. Check with your instructor for variations of the procedure to adapt it to the practice in your area. Place a check mark (✓) in the box as you complete each step.

Steps for Transcribing a Neurodiagnostics Order

1. Read the order. ❑

2. Obtain the Kardex form and requisition form if using the requisition method. ❑

3. Order the study from the neurodiagnostics department. ❑

Use the computer method by:
a. selecting Enter Orders on the master screen ❑
b. selecting the patient's name from the census on the viewing screen ❑
c. selecting the neurodiagnostics department from the department menu on the viewing screen ❑
d. typing in the pertinent data (refer to your patient's MAR)—enter any anticonvulsive medications your patient is taking on the computer screen ❑
e. entering the study to be performed ❑
f. writing "ord" in ink above each order on the doctors' order sheet to indicate that the study has been ordered ❑
g. sending the order by pressing "enter" on the computer keyboard ❑

Use the requisition method by:
a. labeling the neurodiagnostics requisition with patient ID label ❑
b. writing in the pertinent information (refer to your patient's MAR)—write any anticonvulsive medications that your patient is taking on the requisition ❑
c. placing a check mark (✓) in the box next to the study to be ordered ❑
d. writing "ord" in ink above each order on the doctors' order sheet to indicate that the study has been ordered ❑
e. sending the requisition ❑

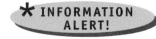
★ INFORMATION ALERT!

It is important for the neurologist who is interpreting the results of the study to know whether the patient is taking an anticonvulsive medication or a medication for sedation. Refer to Chapter 13 in *Health Unit Coordinating*, 5th ed., for a list of these medications. Enter any anticonvulsive medication into the computer or write them on the requisition.

4. Kardex the order by:
   a. writing the date and order in pencil in the diagnostic studies column on the Kardex form ❑
   b. writing in pencil the date that the neurodiagnostics order will be done in the column
      next to the order ❑
   c. writing the symbol "K" in ink in front of the order on the doctors' order sheet to indicate
      completion of the kardexing step ❑
5. Recheck each step for accuracy. ❑
6. Sign off the orders to indicate completion of transcription. ❑

Place a check mark (✔) in the box below to indicate that you have completed Activity 16–2.

❑ Transcribe a Neurodiagnostics Order   Date: _____

ACTIVITY 16-3

TRANSCRIBE AN ENDOSCOPY ORDER

Materials Needed   Black ink pen
                        Red ink pen (depending on hospital policy)
                        Pencil
                        Eraser
                        Kardex form used in Activity 16–2
                        Patient ID labels
                        Consent form for procedure
                        Diet requisition
                        Computer and Practice Activity Software for Transcription of Physicians' Orders
                        Telephone

Directions

Refer to Physicians' Order Sheet 16–3 on your patient's chart. Practice transcribing the endoscopy order and the related orders by following the steps below. Check with your instructor for variations of the procedure to adapt it to the practice in your area. Place a check mark (✔) in the box as you complete each step.

Steps for Transcribing an Endoscopy Order

1. Read the orders. ❑
2. Obtain the Kardex form, diet requisition, and consent to procedure form. ❑

> ✱ **INFORMATION ALERT!**
>
> An endoscopy is usually scheduled by the doctor performing the examination. The date and time of the procedure may be included in the doctors' orders. The endoscopy department should be called to verify the schedule. Some hospitals may require the order to be entered into the computer for billing purposes. A consent form is required for an endoscopy procedure. The consent form is usually transcribed onto the Kardex form. Refer to Activity 8–3 for the steps to prepare a consent form.

3. Schedule the endoscopy examination (or verify if scheduled by doctor) by: ❑
   a. calling the endoscopy department to determine the date and time of the procedure ❑

★ INFORMATION ALERT!

Notify the endoscopy department of the patient's name, unit, room number, and diagnosis. The department will inform you of the time the examination is scheduled. Record the information on the Kardex form. A call to the doctor's office to notify the doctor of the time of examination may be necessary.

    b. preparing the consent form and writing "prepared" above the endoscopy order on the order sheet   ❑

4. Enter the order into the computer or send a requisition for billing purposes.   ❑

5. Order the diet change from the dietary department by computer or by using the requisition method. (refer to the dietary activities in Chapter 12 in this manual).   ❑

6. Kardex the order by:
    a. writing the date and order in pencil in the diagnostic studies column on the Kardex form   ❑
    b. writing the scheduled date and time in pencil in the column next to the order   ❑
    c. writing the symbol "K" in ink in front of the order on the doctors' order sheet to indicate that the order has been kardexed   ❑

7. Kardex the NPO order by:
    a. writing the date and order in the diet column on the Kardex form   ❑
    b. writing the symbol "K" in ink in front of the order on the doctors' order sheet to indicate that the diet order has been kardexed   ❑

8. Recheck each step for accuracy.   ❑

9. Sign off the orders to indicate completion of transcription.   ❑

Place a check mark (✔) in the box below to indicate that you have completed Activity 16–3.

❑ Transcribe an Endoscopy Order   Date: _____

ACTIVITY 16-4

TRANSCRIBE A RESPIRATORY CARE DIAGNOSTIC ORDERA

Materials Needed   Black ink pen
        Red ink pen (depending on hospital policy)
        Pencil
        Eraser
        Kardex form used in Activity 16–3
        MAR used in previous chapters
        Patient ID labels (if using the requisition method)
        Respiratory care diagnostics requisition (if using the requisition method)
        Computer and Practice Activity Software for Transcription of Physicians' Orders

Directions

Refer to Physicians' Order Sheet 16–4 in your patient's chart. Practice transcribing the respiratory care diagnostics order by following the steps below. Check with your instructor for variations of the procedure to adapt it to the practice in your area. Place a check mark (✔) in the box as you complete each step.

Steps for Transcribing a Respiratory Care Diagnostics Order

1. Read the order. ❑

2. Obtain the Kardex form and requisition if using the requisition method. ❑

3. Order the study from the respiratory care department.

Use the computer method by:
a. selecting Enter Orders on the master screen ❑
b. selecting the patient's name from the census on the viewing screen ❑
c. selecting the respiratory care department from the department menu on the viewing screen ❑
d. selecting the diagnostics division from the viewing screen ❑
e. typing in the pertinent information (refer to your patient's MAR)—enter any medications that your patient is taking onto the order screen ❑
f. entering the study to be performed ❑
g. writing "ord" in ink above each order on the doctors' order sheet to indicate that the study has been ordered ❑
h. sending the order by pressing "enter" on the computer keyboard ❑

Use the requisition method by:
a. labeling the respiratory care requisition with patient ID label ❑
b. writing in the pertinent information (refer to your patient's MAR)—write any anticoagulant medications that your patient is taking on the requisition ❑
c. placing a check mark (✓) in the box next to the respiratory care order ❑
d. writing "ord" in ink above each order on the doctors' order sheet to indicate that the studies has been ordered ❑
e. sending the requisition ❑

★ INFORMATION ALERT!

The respiratory care department performs both diagnostic tests and treatments. Some hospitals call this department the cardiopulmonary department.

4. Kardex the order by: ❑
a. writing the date and order in pencil in the pulmonary function column on the Kardex form ❑
b. writing the symbol "K" in ink in front of the respiratory care order on the doctors' order sheet to indicate completion of the kardexing step ❑

5. Recheck each step for accuracy. ❑

6. Sign off the order to indicate completion of transcription. ❑

Place a check mark (✔) in the box below to indicate that you have completed Activity 16–4.

❑ Transcribe a Respiratory Care Diagnostics Order   Date: _____

ACTIVITY 16-5

TRANSCRIBE A REVIEW SET OF DOCTORS' ORDERS

Materials Needed   Black ink pen

Red ink pen (depending on hospital policy)

Pencil

Eraser

Kardex form used in Activity 16–4

MAR used in Activity 16–4

Patient ID labels

All necessary forms

Computer and Practice Activity Software for Transcription of Physicians' Orders

Directions

Refer to Physicians' Order Sheet 16–5 in your patient's chart. Transcribe the orders. Refer to previous activities for the appropriate steps as needed.

Steps for Transcribing a Review Set of Doctors' Orders

1. Read the orders.   ❏
2. Send or fax pharmacy copy to pharmacy.   ❏
3. Check orders for stats.   ❏
4. Make any necessary telephone calls.   ❏
5. Obtain all necessary forms.   ❏

Suggestion to the student: Use this space to list the forms you will need.

6. Order as necessary.   ❏
7. Prepare consent forms as required.   ❏
8. Kardex the orders.   ❏
9. Record the medications on the MAR.   ❏
10. Recheck each step for accuracy.   ❏
11. Sign off the orders to indicate completion of transcription.   ❏

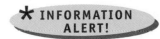

✱ INFORMATION ALERT!

Transcribing doctors' orders is a critical task, and an error could cause harm to a patient. If you are not absolutely sure in interpreting the doctors' orders, ask the patient's nurse or the doctor who wrote the orders.

Place a check mark (✔) in the box below to indicate that you have completed Activity 16–5.

☐ Transcribe a Review Set of Doctors' Orders   Date: _____

ACTIVITY 16-6
RECORD TELEPHONED DOCTORS' ORDERS

Materials Needed   Pen
                          Physicians' order sheet

Directions

Practice recording the telephoned physicians' orders printed below by following the steps below. Place a check mark (✔) in the box as you complete each step.

Telephoned Physicians' Orders

"Hello, this is Dr. Hart with orders on John Smith—ready?

Complete bed rest

Vital signs every 4 hours until stable

If systolic blood pressure is over 190, call the house officer

Low-sodium, low-residue diet

Start 1000 cubic centimeters of 5% dextrose in lactated Ringer's to keep open

Twelve-lead electrocardiogram—clinical indication: cardiac arrhythmia

Electroencephalogram—clinical indication: rule out seizer activity

Arterial blood gases on room air—please call me with results; my back office number is 555-3245

Notify Mr. Smith's family that I will be at the hospital about 8 o'clock this evening. Thanks."

Steps for Transcribing Physicians' Orders

1. Have someone read the above orders to you while you record them on a physicians' order sheet.   ☐

2. Use accepted abbreviations and symbols as you write the orders.   ☐

3. For further practice, obtain a new Kardex and practice transcribing the orders you have written.   ☐

Place a check mark (✔) in the box below to indicate that you have completed Activity 16–6.

☐ Record Telephoned Doctors' Orders   Date: _____

ACTIVITY 16-6

RECORD TELEPHONE MESSAGES

Materials Needed   Pen or pencil
Message pad

Directions

Practice recording the telephone messages printed below by following the steps below. Place a check mark (✓) in the box as you complete each step.

Telephone Messages

1. "Hello, this is Jane in the cardiovascular lab. Would you check Mary Copa's medication record and tell me what medications she is taking and check the nurse's admission record for a weight and height. Someone forgot to note this information on the requisition. Thanks."   ❏

2. "Hi, this is Pete in endoscopy. Please ask John Smith's nurse to give the on-call medication now. We will be up to get him in twenty minutes, please have his chart ready. Thanks."   ❏

Steps for Recording Telephone Messages

1. Have someone read the above messages to you while you record them on a message pad.   ❏

2. Write down who the message is for.   ❏

3. Write down the caller's name.   ❏

4. Write down the date and time of the call.   ❏

5. Write down the purpose of the call.   ❏

6. If a return call is expected, write down the number to call.   ❏

7. Sign your name to the message.   ❏

Place a check mark (✔) in the box below to indicate that you have completed Activity 16–7.

❏ Record Telephone Messages   Date: _____

PHYSICIANS' ORDER SHEET 16–1

DATE	TIME	SYMBOL	ORDERS
			EKG c̄ rhythm strip now
			Treadmill stress test in am } poss occlusion
			Dr

PHYSICIANS' ORDER SHEET 16–2

DATE	TIME	SYMBOL	ORDERS
			EEG to evaluate seizure activity
			AER to evaluate hearing loss
			Dr

PHYSICIANS' ORDER SHEET 16–3

DATE	TIME	SYMBOL	ORDERS
			Esophagoscopy @ 0800 in AM
			NPO 2400 hrs
			Have consent signed per Dr John Peppercorn
			Dr

PHYSICIANS' ORDER SHEET 16–4

DATE	TIME	SYMBOL	ORDERS
			Spirometry today
			ABG on RA—page hospitalist c̄ results
			Dr

PHYSICIANS' ORDER SHEET 16–5

DATE	TIME	SYMBOL	ORDERS
			Advance DAT
			Amb c̄ help bid
			2D M mode echo poss occlusion
			Repeat ABG now
			Chest PA & LAT Cl: valley fever
			Cardiac enzymes & CNP now
			CMP in AM
			Sputum for AFB Cx & stain
			DC IV & convert to heplock c̄ rout saline flushes
			Dr
			Heart catheterization at 0930 per Dr. Joseph Packer
			Valium 20 mg IM on call to cath lab
			Dr

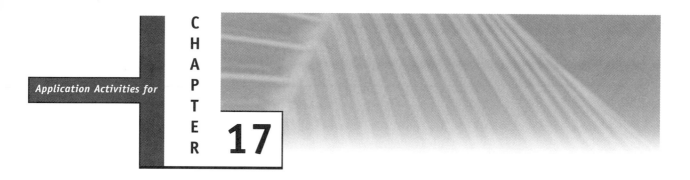

Treatment Orders

Place the Physicians' Order Sheets located at the end of the chapter in your patient's chart. Follow the directions for each activity to transcribe orders.

Activities in This Chapter

Transcribe
17–1: Traction Orders
17–2: Respiratory Care Orders
17–3: Physical Medicine and Rehabilitation Orders
17–4: A Review Set of Doctors' Orders

Record
17–5: Telephoned Doctors' Orders
17–6: Telephone Messages

ACTIVITY 17-1

TRANSCRIBE TRACTION ORDERS

Materials Needed

Black ink pen

Red ink pen (depending on hospital policy)

Pencil

Eraser

Kardex form used in previous chapters

Patient ID labels (if using requisition method)

CSD requisition

Computer and Practice Activity Software for Transcription of Physicians' Orders

Directions

Refer to Physicians' Order Sheet 17–1 in your patient's chart. Practice transcribing the traction orders by following the steps below. Check with your instructor for variations of the procedure to adapt it to the practice in your area. Place a check mark (✓) in the box as you complete each step.

Steps for Transcribing Traction Orders

1. Read the orders. ❑

2. Obtain the Kardex form and requisition form if using the requisition method. ❑

3. Order the orthopedic equipment from the central service department.

Use the computer method by:
a. selecting Enter Orders on the master screen ❑
b. selecting the patient's name from the census on the viewing screen ❑
c. selecting the orthopedic equipment department from the department menu on the viewing screen ❑
d. typing in the pertinent information ❑
e. selecting the orthopedic equipment to be ordered from the menu on the viewing screen ❑
f. writing "ord" in ink in front of the order on the doctors' order sheet to indicate that the orthopedic equipment has been ordered ❑
g. sending the order by pressing "enter" on the computer keyboard ❑

Use the requisition method by:
a. labeling the orthopedic equipment requisition with patient ID label ❑
b. writing in the pertinent information ❑
c. placing a check mark (✓) in the box next to the equipment to be ordered ❑
d. writing "ord" in ink above each order on the doctor's order sheet to indicate that the orthopedic equipment has been ordered ❑
e. sending the requisition ❑

4. Notify the patient's nurse verbally of the order and document the name of the nurse with the time notified above the order on the physicians' order sheet. ❑

5. Kardex the orders by:
a. writing the date and order in pencil in the treatment column on the Kardex form ❑
b. writing the symbol "K" in ink in front of the order on the doctors' order sheet to indicate completion of the kardexing step ❑

6. Recheck each step for accuracy. ❑

7. Sign off the orders to indicate completion of transcription. ❑

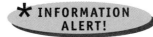

To transcribe a doctor's order to discontinue traction, notify the patient's nurse or the orthopedic technician (if employed at that hospital) by telephone. Record "notified" or "called" and the time next to the order on the doctors' order sheet to indicate the completion of the transcription step. When using a computer, enter the discontinued order into the computer.

Place a check mark (✓) in the box below to indicate that you have completed Activity 17–1.

 Transcribe Traction Orders   Date: _____

ACTIVITY 17-2

TRANSCRIBE RESPIRATORY CARE ORDERS

Materials Needed   Black ink pen
Red ink pen (depending on hospital policy)
Pencil
Eraser

Kardex form used in Activity 17–1

Patient ID labels (if using requisition method)

Respiratory care requisition

Computer and Practice Activity Software for Transcription of Physicians' Orders

Directions

Refer to Physicians' Order Sheet 17–2 in your patient's chart. Practice transcribing the respiratory care orders by following the steps below. Check with your instructor for variations of the procedure to adapt it to the practice in your area. Place a check mark (✓) in the box as you complete each step.

Steps for Transcribing Respiratory Care Order

1. Read the orders. ❑

2. Obtain the Kardex form and respiratory care department requisition if using the requisition method. ❑

3. Order the respiratory treatment(s) and equipment from the respiratory care department.

Use the computer method by:
a. selecting Enter Orders on the master screen ❑
b. selecting the patient's name from the census on the viewing screen ❑
c. selecting the respiratory care department from the department menu on the viewing screen ❑
d. selecting the appropriate division from the respiratory care divisions screen ❑
e. typing in the pertinent information ❑
f. selecting treatment(s) and equipment to be ordered from the menu on the screen ❑
g. writing "ord" in ink above each order on the doctor's order sheet to indicate that the treatment(s) and equipment has (have) been ordered ❑
h. sending the order by pressing "enter" on the computer keyboard ❑

Use the requisition method by:
a. labeling the respiratory care department requisition with patient ID label ❑
b. writing in the pertinent information ❑
c. placing a check mark (✓) in the box next to the respiratory treatment(s) and equipment to be ordered (writing any special instructions in the space provided) ❑
d. writing "ord" in ink above each order on the doctors' order sheet to indicate that the respiratory treatment(s) or equipment has (have) been ordered ❑
e. sending the requisition ❑

✱ INFORMATION ALERT!

Medications such as Vaponefrin, Mucomyst, Decadron, Bronkosol, terbutaline, Alupent, albuterol, and Vanceril are commonly used with respiratory treatments. It may be the responsibility of either the health unit coordinator (send pharmacy copy or fax orders) or the respiratory therapist to order the medication.

4. Kardex the orders by:
a. writing the date and order in pencil in the respiratory care column on the Kardex form ❑
b. writing the symbol "K" in ink in front of the order on the doctors' order sheet to indicate completion of the kardexing step ❑

5. Recheck each step for accuracy. ❑

6. Sign off the orders to indicate completion of transcription. To transcribe a doctors' order to discontinue respiratory care, enter the discontinued order into the computer. It may be necessary to notify the respiratory care department by telephone. Record "called" and the time called next to the order on the doctors' order sheet to indicate the completion of the transcription step. ❑

Place a check mark (✔) in the box below to indicate that you have completed Activity 17–2.

☐ Transcribe Respiratory Care Orders   Date: _____

ACTIVITY 17-3

TRANSCRIBE PHYSICAL MEDICINE AND REHABILITATION ORDERS

Materials Needed   Black ink pen

Red ink pen (depending on hospital policy)

Pencil

Eraser

Kardex form used in Activity 17–2

Patient ID labels (if using requisition method)

Physical medicine and rehabilitation requisition

Computer and Practice Activity Software for Transcription of Physicians' Orders

Directions

Refer to Physicians' Order Sheet 17–3 in your patient's chart. Practice transcribing the physical medicine and rehabilitation orders by following the steps below. Check with your instructor for variations of the procedure to adapt it to the practice in your area. Place a check mark (✔) in the box as you complete each step.

Steps for Transcribing Physical Medicine and Rehabilitation Orders

1. Read the orders.   ☐

2. Obtain the Kardex form and requisition(s) if using the requisition method.   ☐

★ INFORMATION ALERT!

Each order may require a separate requisition, as each may be performed by a different division in the physical medicine and rehabilitation department.

3. Order the physical medicine or rehabilitation treatment(s) from the physical medicine and   ☐
rehabilitation department.

Use the computer method by:
a. selecting Enter Orders on the master screen   ☐
b. selecting the patient's name from the census on the viewing screen   ☐
c. selecting the physical medicine department from the department menu on the   ☐
   viewing screen
d. selecting the appropriate division in the physical medicine department   ☐
e. typing in the pertinent information   ☐
f. entering the complete order   ☐
g. writing "ord" above each order on the doctor's order sheet to indicate that the physical   ☐
   medicine or rehabilitation treatment has been ordered
h. sending the order by pressing "enter" on the computer keyboard   ☐

Use the requisition method by:
a. labeling the physical medicine requisitions with patient ID label   ☐
b. writing in the pertinent information   ☐
c. writing the complete order(s) in the appropriate space on the requisition   ☐

d. writing "ord" in ink above each order on the doctors' order sheet to indicate that the physical medicine or rehabilitation treatments have been ordered ☐

e. sending the requisition ☐

4. Kardex the orders by:

a. writing the date and order in pencil in the physical medicine column on the Kardex form ☐

b. writing the symbol "K" in ink in front of the order on the doctors' order sheet to indicate completion of the kardexing step ☐

5. Recheck each step for accuracy. ☐

6. Sign off the orders to indicate completion of transcription. ☐

✱ INFORMATION ALERT!

To transcribe a doctors' order to discontinue physical medicine or rehabilitation treatments, enter the discontinued order into the computer.

Place a check mark (✔) in the box below to indicate that you have completed Activity 17–3.

☐ Transcribe Physical Medicine and Rehabilitation Orders   Date: _____

ACTIVITY 17-4

TRANSCRIBE A REVIEW SET OF DOCTORS' ORDERS

Materials Needed

Black ink pen

Red ink pen (depending on hospital policy)

Pencil

Eraser

Kardex form used in Activity 17–3

MAR used in previous chapters

Patient ID labels (if using requisition method)

All necessary forms

Computer and Practice Activity Software for Transcription of Physicians' Orders

Directions

Refer to Physicians' Order Sheet 17–4 in your patient's chart. Transcribe the orders. Refer to previous activities for the appropriate steps as needed.

Steps for Transcribing a Review Set of Doctors' Orders

1. Read the orders. ☐

2. Send pharmacy copy or fax orders to pharmacy. ☐

3. Check orders for stats. ☐

4. Place any necessary phone calls. ☐

5. Obtain all necessary forms. ☐

6. Order as necessary. ☐

Suggestion to the student: Use this space to list the forms you will need.

7. Kardex the orders. ☐

8. Record the medications on the MAR. ☐

9. Recheck each step for accuracy. ☐

10. Sign off the orders to indicate completion of transcription. ☐

✱ INFORMATION ALERT!

Transcribing doctors' orders is a critical task, and an error could cause harm to a patient. If you are not absolutely sure in interpreting the doctors' orders, ask the patient's nurse or the doctor who wrote the orders.

Place a check mark (✓) in the box below to indicate that you have completed Activity 17–4.

☐ Transcribe a Review Set of Doctors' Orders   Date: _____

ACTIVITY 17-5

RECORD TELEPHONED DOCTORS' ORDERS

Materials Needed   Pen
                             Physicians' order sheet

Directions

Practice recording the telephoned doctors' orders printed below by following the steps below. Place a check mark (✓) in the box as you complete each step.

Telephoned Physicians' Orders

"Hello, this is Dr. Ted Smith with orders on John Brown.

Discontinue the whirlpool baths

Physical therapy to start active assistance exercises to bilateral lower extremities three times a day

Discontinue oxygen

Monitored dose inhaler with Ventolin two puffs four times a day

Hot packs to lumbar spine twice a day

Demerol 50 or 100 milligrams every 3–4 hours as necessary for pain

Thank you."

Steps for Transcribing Physicians' Orders

1. Have someone read the above orders to you while you record them on a doctor's order
sheet. ❑

2. Use accepted abbreviations and symbols as you write the orders. ❑

3. For further practice, obtain a new Kardex and practice transcribing the orders you
have written. ❑

Place a check mark (✔) in the box below to indicate that you have completed Activity 17–5.

❑ Record Telephoned Doctors' Orders   Date: _____

ACTIVITY 17-6
RECORD TELEPHONE MESSAGES

Materials Needed   Pen or pencil
Message pad

Directions

Practice recording the telephone messages printed below by following the steps below. Place a check mark (✔) in the box
as you complete each step.

Telephone Messages

1. "Hi, this is Hal in physical therapy. We would like to bring Mary Copa down for her whirlpool
at 2:00 PM. Would you check with her nurse to see if that time is OK? Thanks."

2. "Hello, this is June in the recovery room. Please tell John Smith's nurse that John is now in
the recovery room. Have gastric suction and oxygen set up in his room. I will call when he
is ready to return to the unit. Thanks."

Steps for Recording Telephone Messages

1. Have someone read the preceding messages to you while you record them on a message pad. ❑

2. Write down who the message is for. ❑

3. Write down the caller's name. ❑

4. Write down the date and time of the call ❑

5. Write down the purpose of the call. ❑

6. If a return call is expected, write down the number to call. ❑

7. Sign your name to the message. ❑

Place a check mark (✔) in the box below to indicate that you have completed Activity 17–6.

❑ Record Telephone Messages   Date: _____

PHYSICIANS' ORDER SHEET 17–1

DATE	TIME	SYMBOL	ORDERS
			Bucks tx 10# to lt leg
			Overhead frame & trapeze
			Dr

PHYSICIANS' ORDER SHEET 17–2

DATE	TIME	SYMBOL	ORDERS
			O_2 4 L/M N/P
			SVN 0.5 cc Albuterol in 2 cc NS q 4° c̄ CPT
			Induced sputum specimen for C & S
			Dr
			D/C Bucks tx
			Dr

PHYSICIANS' ORDER SHEET 17–3

DATE	TIME	SYMBOL	ORDERS
			Crutch training WBAT lt leg
			US & ES to lt leg bid
			Rom lt leg bid
			OT for eval & tx
			Dr

PHYSICIANS' ORDER SHEET 17–4

DATE	TIME	SYMBOL	ORDERS
			Reg diet—FF
			Apical pulse c̄ VS q 4°
			orthostatic B/P tid
			Carotid US CI: UE numbness
			EEG to eval. cause of H/As
			2 D M mode echo CI: UE numbness
			ESR & BUN & creatinine
			△ synthroid to 125 mcg po daily
			Dulcolax ī po q pm
			Insert picc and start IV of 1000 cc 0.45 NS c̄ 40 meq KCL 12
			Strict I & O
			Daily wt @ 0700
			Dr
			MUGA scan
			stat lytes & call c̄ results
			D/C O₂
			△ ROM lt leg to qd
			△ Change SVN to q 6°
			Dr

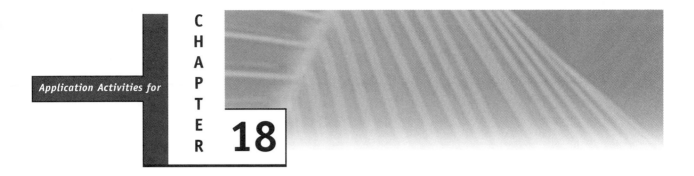

Application Activities for

C
H
A
P
T
E
R
18

Miscellaneous Orders

Place the Physicians' Order Sheets located at the end of the chapter in your patient's chart. Follow the directions for each activity to transcribe orders.

Activities in This Chapter

Transcribe

ACTIVITY 18-1

TRANSCRIBE A CONSULTATION ORDER

Materials Needed   Black ink pen

Red ink pen (depending on hospital policy)

Pencil

Eraser

Telephone

Simulated doctors' roster provided in the Practice Activity Software for Transcription of Physicians' Orders or by your instructor

Kardex form used in previous chapters

Situation

You are the health unit coordinator on 5W, a cardiovascular unit, at College Hospital. Your patient's doctor writes a consultation order for a patient.

Directions

Refer to Physicians' Order Sheet 18–1 in your patient's chart. Practice transcribing the consultation order using the above situation. Follow the steps below. Check with your instructor for variations of the procedure to adapt it to the practice in your area. Place a check mark (✓) in the box as you complete each step.

Steps for Transcribing a Consultation Order

1. Read the order. ❑

2. Record the following information on your note pad. ❑

NOTE PAD

Consulting doctor's name and telephone number: _____

Hospital name: _____

Patient's name: _____

Patient's location (unit and room number): _____

Name of the doctor requesting the consultation: _____

Patient's diagnosis: _____

---

3. Communicate the order by:
   a. telephoning the doctor's office or answering service using the information in step 2 ❑
   b. writing "called" and the name or operator number of the person you spoke to and the time you called in ink above the order or in the right margin on the doctors' order sheet to indicate the doctor's office has been notified ❑

4. Obtain the Kardex form and simulated doctors' roster. ❑

5. Kardex the order by:
   a. writing the date and order in pencil in the consultation column on the Kardex form ❑
   b. writing the symbol "K" in ink in front of the order on the doctors' order sheet to indicate completion of the kardexing step ❑

6. Recheck each step for accuracy. ❑

7. Sign off the order to indicate completion of transcription. ❑

★ INFORMATION ALERT!

On some hospital units, physicians are required or may wish to call the consulting physician themselves so that a patient history and other information may be given.

Place a check mark (✔) in the box below to indicate that you have completed Activity 18–1.

❑ Transcribe a Consultation Order   Date: _____

ACTIVITY 18-2

TRANSCRIBE A HEALTH RECORDS ORDER

Materials Needed   Black ink pen
Red ink pen (depending on hospital policy)
Pencil
Eraser
Kardex form used in Activity 18–1
Telephone

Directions

Refer to Physicians' Order Sheet 18–2 in your patient's chart. Practice transcribing the order for obtaining the health records by following the steps below. Check with your instructor for variations of the procedure to adapt it to the practice in your area. Place a check mark (✓) in the box as you complete each step.

Steps for Transcribing a Health Records Order

1. Read the order. ❏

2. Communicate the order by:
   a. telephoning the health records department to request that the records of the patient be sent to your unit ❏
   b. writing "called" and the name of the person you spoke to and the time you called in ink above the order or in the right margin on the doctors' order sheet to indicate that the health records have been requested ❏

3. Obtain the Kardex form. ❏

4. Kardex the order by:
   a. placing a check mark (✓) and the date next to "Health Records" or recording the information on the Kardex form ❏
   b. Writing the symbol "K" in ink in front of the order on the doctors' order sheet to indicate completion of the kardexing step ❏

5. Recheck each step for accuracy. ❏

6. Sign off the order to indicate completion of transcription. ❏

✻ INFORMATION ALERT!

In the hospital setting, the doctor may request records from the patient's previous stay in another hospital. Because the information is confidential, you must prepare a consent form to be signed by the patient. The consent form will then be faxed to the health records department of the other hospital. The records will be released and faxed to your unit.

Place a check mark (✔) in the box below to indicate that you have completed Activity 18–2.

❏ Transcribe a Health Records Order   Date: _____

ACTIVITY 18-3

TRANSCRIBE AN ORDER FOR CASE MANAGEMENT

Materials Needed
Black ink pen
Red ink pen (depending on hospital policy)
Pencil
Eraser
Note pad
Kardex form used in Activity 18–2
Telephone
Computer and Practice Activity Software for Transcription of Physicians' Orders

Directions

Refer to Physicians' Order Sheet 18–3 in your patient's chart. Practice transcribing the order for case management by following the steps below. Check with your instructor for variations of the procedure to adapt it to the practice in your area. Place a check mark (✓) in the box as you complete each step.

Steps for Transcribing an Order for Case Management

1. Read the order. ❏

2. Communicate the order by:
   a. entering the order into the computer or by telephoning the case manager assigned to the patient to relay the doctor's written order ❏
   b. writing "called," the name of the person you spoke to, the time you called, and your initials in ink above the order or in the right margin on the doctors' order sheet to indicate that the case manager was notified ❏

3. Obtain the Kardex form. ❏

4. Kardex the order by:
   a. writing the date and the order in the appropriate area on the Kardex ❏
   b. writing the symbol "K" in ink in front of the order on the doctors' order sheet to indicate completion of the kardexing step ❏

5. Recheck each step for accuracy. ❏

6. Sign off the order to indicate completion of transcription. ❏

> ★ **INFORMATION ALERT!**
>
> Case managers work out of the social service department. Some patients are not assigned a case manager, and the social worker will provide support services to the patient and/or family.

Place a check mark (✓) in the box below to indicate that you have completed Activity 18–3.

❏ Transcribe an order for case management   Date: _____

ACTIVITY 18-4

TRANSCRIBE AN ORDER TO SCHEDULE AN EXAMINATION

Materials Needed   Black ink pen

Red ink pen (depending on hospital policy)

Pencil

Eraser

Note pad

Kardex form used in Activity 18–3

Telephone

Directions

Refer to Physicians' Order Sheet 18–4 in your patient's chart. Practice transcribing the order to schedule the examination by following the steps below. Check with your instructor for variations of the procedure to adapt it to the practice in your area. Place a check mark (✓) in the box as you complete each step.

Steps for Transcribing an Order to Schedule an Examination

1. Read the order. ❑

2. Schedule the examination by:
   a. telephoning the appropriate department to arrange an appointment ❑
   b. writing "called," time of appointment, and the name of the person you spoke to and the time in ink above the order or in the right margin on the doctors' order sheet to indicate that the examination has been scheduled ❑

3. Obtain the Kardex form. ❑

4. Kardex the order by:
   a. writing the date and scheduled time and date of the appointment in pencil in the appropriate column on the Kardex form ❑
   b. writing the symbol "K" in ink in front of the order on the doctors' order sheet to indicate completion of the kardexing step ❑

5. Recheck each step for accuracy. ❑

6. Sign off the order to indicate completion of transcription. ❑

Place a check mark (✓) in the box below to indicate that you have completed Activity 18–4.

❑ Transcribe an Order to Schedule an Examination   Date: _____

ACTIVITY 18-5

TRANSCRIBE A REVIEW SET OF DOCTORS' ORDERS

Materials Needed   Black ink pen

Red ink pen (depending on hospital policy)

Pencil

Eraser

Kardex form used in Activity 18–4

MAR used in previous chapters

Telephone

Patient ID labels

All necessary forms

Computer and Practice Activity Software for Transcription of Physicians' Orders

Directions

Refer to Physicians' Order Sheet 18–5 in your patient's chart. Transcribe the orders. Refer to previous activities for the appropriate steps as needed.

Steps for Transcribing a Review Set of Doctors' Orders

1. Read the orders.   ❏
2. Send the pharmacy copy or fax doctors' orders to the pharmacy.   ❏
3. Check orders for stats.   ❏
4. Place telephone calls.   ❏
5. Obtain all necessary forms.   ❏

Suggestion to the student: Use this space to list the forms you will need.

---

6. Order as necessary.   ❏
7. Kardex the orders.   ❏
8. Record the medications on the MAR.   ❏
9. Recheck each step for accuracy.   ❏
10. Sign off the orders to indicate completion of transcription.   ❏

✱ INFORMATION ALERT!

Transcribing doctors' orders is a critical task, and an error could cause harm to a patient. If you are not absolutely sure in interpreting the doctors' orders, ask the patient's nurse or the doctor who wrote them.

Place a check mark (✔) in the box below to indicate that you have completed Activity 18–5.

❏ Transcribe a Review Set of Doctors' Orders   Date: _____

✱ INFORMATION ALERT!

When you have completed Activity 18–5, take all the forms out of your chart. Your patient has been discharged! Your instructor will advise you of proper procedure in preparing patient's chart for health records. Refer to Chapter 20 in *Health Unit Coordinating*, 5th ed.

PHYSICIANS' ORDER SHEET 18–1

DATE	TIME	SYMBOL	ORDERS
			Dr. Ted Johnson for cardiovascular consult ASAP
			Dr

PHYSICIANS' ORDER SHEET 18–2

DATE	TIME	SYMBOL	ORDERS
			Obtain medical records from admission 5 years ago
			to this hospital
			Thank you,
			Dr

PHYSICIANS' ORDER SHEET 18–3

DATE	TIME	SYMBOL	ORDERS
			Case management to arrange for long-term care
			Dr

PHYSICIANS' ORDER SHEET 18–4

DATE	TIME	SYMBOL	ORDERS
			Schedule patient to start radiation therapy c̄ Valley Radiology
			1 wk p̄ DC.
			Dr

PHYSICIANS' ORDER SHEET 18–5

DATE	TIME	SYMBOL	ORDERS
			Up ad-lib c̄ crutches
			Chest PA & LAT Cl:√ for infiltrates
			CBC & BMP today—call c̄ results
			Ua this am
			EKG-LOC today
			Obtain dictated hearth cath report from health records
			D/C ES & US
			D/C ROM exercises
			D/C O$_2$ then do ABG's in 2°
			pt to be transferred to Williams Rehab Center in am
			Please copy & send last 2 days lab & xray results & nursing
			& progress notes c̄ patient
			Dr
			Please have social services arrange for transportation
			Dr

Health Unit Coordinator Procedures

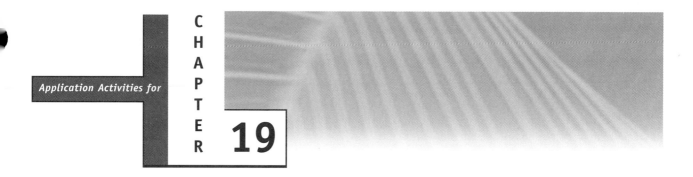

Application Activities for

CHAPTER 19

Admission, Preoperative, and Postoperative Procedures

Place the Physicians' Order Sheets located at the end of the chapter in your patient's chart. Follow the directions for each activity to transcribe orders.

Activities in This Chapter

19–1: Admit a Patient to a Nursing Unit

Transcribe:
19–2: A Set of Admission Orders
19–3: A Set of Preoperative Orders
19–4: A Set of Postoperative Orders

ACTIVITY 19-1

ADMIT A PATIENT TO A NURSING UNIT

Materials Needed
Black ink pen
Red ink pen (depending on hospital policy)
Pencil
Eraser
New Kardex form
New medication record
Patient ID labels
Standard admission chart forms
Daily census sheet
Admission service agreement form
Computer and Practice Activity Software for Transcription of Physicians' Orders
Front sheet

Situation

A patient is being admitted to your unit at Opportunity Medical Center with a diagnosis of "degenerative arthritis." The patient arrives on your unit with an admission service agreement form, a front sheet, and the patient ID labels that have been prepared by the admitting department.

Directions

Place the standard chart forms in your patient's chart. Practice the health unit coordinator task to admit a patient to your unit using the information in the above situation. Ask another student to role-play when necessary in the steps below. Check with your instructor for variations of the procedure to adapt it to the practice in your area. Place a check mark (✓) in the box as you complete each step.

Steps for Admitting a Patient to a Nursing Unit

1. Greet the patient upon arrival at the nurses' station. ❏

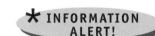

Introduce yourself and give your status. Example: "I am (*your name*), the health unit coordinator for this unit." Some hospitals have added bedside admitting responsibilities to the health unit coordinator. In this case the health unit coordinator would go to the patient's bedside and enter admitting information given by patient into a laptop computer.

2. Notify the nurse of the patient's arrival and inform the patient that you have notified the nurse. ❏

3. Record the patient's admission on the census sheet and enter the information into the computer if available. ❏

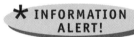

Add the patient's name to the census using the computer by selecting the Admission screen, then filling in the pertinent information.

4. Check the patient's signature on the admission service agreement form. ❏

5. If using the computer and Practice Activity Software for Transcription of Physicians' Orders, follow the directions provided in the software and admit a patient (make up a name) using a doctor from the physicians roster provided in the software. ❏

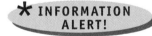

Compare the spelling of the patient's name on the front sheet and the ID labels. When possible also check the spelling with the patient's signature and on the insurance card. Check to see that the doctor's name is correct.

6. Complete the procedure for the preparation of the chart forms. (Refer to Activity 8–2). ❏

7. Place the patient ID labels in your patient's chart. ❏

8. Label and fill in the necessary information on the patient's Kardex form and MAR to be found in Appendix B. ❏

9. Place the allergy information (usually obtained from the nurse's admission notes and doctors' orders) on the front of the patient's chart, the Kardex form, and the MAR. Prepare an allergy bracelet for the patient if necessary. ❏

10. Notify the attending doctor and/or the hospital resident of the patient's admission. ❏

Place a check mark (✓) in the box below to indicate that you have completed Activity 19–1.

❏ Admit a Patient to a Nursing Unit   Date: _____

ACTIVITY 19-2

TRANSCRIBE A SET OF ADMISSION ORDERS

Materials Needed   Black ink pen

Red ink pen (depending on hospital policy)

Pencil

Eraser

Admission order form used in Skills Activity 19–1

Kardex form used in Skills Activity 19–1

MAR used in Skills Activity 19–1

Telephone

Patient ID labels

All necessary forms

Computer and Practice Activity Software for Transcription of Physicians' Orders

Directions

Refer to Physicians' Order Sheet 19–2 in your patient's chart. Transcribe the orders. Refer to previous activities for the appropriate steps as needed.

Steps for Transcribing a Set of Admission Orders

1. Read the orders.   ❏

2. Send the pharmacy copy of the orders or fax the orders to pharmacy.   ❏

3. Check orders for stats.   ❏

4. Place telephone calls.   ❏

5. Obtain all necessary forms.   ❏

6. Order as necessary, using the computer or requisition method.   ❏

7. Kardex the orders.   ❏

8. Record the medications on the MAR.   ❏

Suggestion to the student: Use this space to list the forms you will need.

9. Recheck each step for accuracy. ❑

10. Sign off the orders to indicate completion of transcription. ❑

Place a check mark (✔) in the box below to indicate that you have completed Activity 19–2.

❑ Transcribe a Set of Admission Orders　　　　Date: _____

ACTIVITY 19-3
TRANSCRIBE A SET OF PREOPERATIVE ORDERS

Materials Needed　　Black ink pen
Red ink pen (depending on hospital policy)
Pencil
Eraser
Kardex form used in Activity 19–2
MAR used in Activity 19–2
Telephone
Patient ID labels
All necessary forms
Computer and Practice Activity Software for Transcription of Physicians' Orders

Directions

Refer to Physicians' Order Sheet 19–3 in your patient's chart. This order form contains two sets of preoperative orders. Transcribe each set separately. Refer to previous activities for the appropriate steps as needed.

Steps for Transcribing a Set of Preoperative Orders

1. Read the orders. ❑

2. Send the pharmacy copy of the orders or fax the orders to pharmacy. ❑

3. Check orders for stats. ❑

Suggestion to the student: Use this space to list the forms you will need.

4. Place telephone calls. ❏

5. Obtain all necessary forms. ❏

6. Order as necessary, using the computer or requisition method. ❏

7. Kardex the orders. ❏

8. Record the medications on the MAR. ❏

9. Recheck all orders for accuracy. ❏

10. Sign off the orders to indicate completion of transcription. ❏

Place a check mark (✔) in the box below to indicate that you have completed Activity 19–3.

❏ Transcribe a Set of Preoperative Orders   Date: _____

ACTIVITY 19-4

TRANSCRIBE A SET OF POSTOPERATIVE ORDERS

Materials Needed   Black ink pen

Red ink pen (depending on hospital policy)

Pencil

Eraser

New Kardex form

New medication record

Telephone

Patient ID labels

All necessary forms

Computer and Practice Activity Software for Transcription of Physicians' Orders

Directions

Refer to Physicians' Order Sheet 19–4 in your patient's chart. Transcribe the orders. Refer to previous activities for the appropriate steps as needed.

Steps for Transcribing a Set of Postoperative Orders

1. Read the orders. ❑

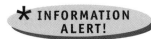

> **★ INFORMATION ALERT!**
>
> All preoperative orders are automatically discontinued postoperatively. The health unit coordinator would obtain a new Kardex form and new MAR. The previous MAR would be placed in the patient's chart under the medication divider. Refer to Chapter 19 in *Health Unit Coordinating*, 5th ed.

2. Send the pharmacy copy of the orders or fax the orders to pharmacy. ❑

3. Check orders for stats. ❑

4. Place telephone calls. ❑

5. Obtain all necessary forms. ❑

6. Order as necessary, using the computer or requisition method. ❑

7. Kardex the orders. ❑

8. Record the medications on the MAR. ❑

9. Recheck all orders for accuracy. ❑

10. Sign off the orders to indicate completion of transcription. ❑

Place a check mark (✔) in the box below to indicate that you have completed Activity 19–4.

❑ Transcribe a Set of Postoperative Orders   Date: _____

Suggestion to the student: Use this space to list the forms you will need.

PHYSICIANS' ORDER SHEET 19–2

DATE	TIME	SYMBOL	ORDERS
			Admit to med surg unit
			DX: Degenerative arthritis
			Allergies: PCN
			CBR c̄ BSC
			VS per rout
			Mech soft diet
			Start IVF of 1000 cc D5LR @ 120 cc/hr
			CBC, PT, PTT today
			CMP in am
			Ua
			Chest PA & Lat Cl: pre-op
			EKG pre-op
			Tylenol ii PO q 4-6° H/A—minor aches
			Demerol 50 or 100 mg IM q 4-6° sev pain
			Notify Dr Joseph Sergen of pts admission
			Valley anesthesia for pre-op orders
			Dr Penny Primery MD

PHYSICIANS' ORDER SHEET 19–3

DATE	TIME	SYMBOL	ORDERS
			Hibiclens bath this pm
			T & X match 2 U PC—hold for surg
			Resp dept to do pre-op teaching
			OH frame & trapeze to bed
			Have consent signed for rt total hip replacement
			Dr Joseph Sergen MD
			Cl liq breakfast @ 0600, then NPO
			Restoril 15 mg PO hs MR x 1 if nec
			Demerol 100 mg ⎫
			Vistaril 25 mg ⎭ IM 1230
			Dr Patrick Snooze MD

PHYSICIANS' ORDER SHEET 19-4

DATE	TIME	SYMBOL	ORDERS
			VS q 2° until stable, then q 4°
			1000 cc D5NS c̄ 20 meq KCL @ 120 cc/hr
			Cl liq to DAT when active bowel sounds present
			Keep hemovac compressed & record drainage q shift
			Strict I & O
			Foley cath to st drainage
			Ted hose thigh high—both legs
			IS q 2 hr
			PT to initiate total hip protocol
			OT consult on 2nd PO day
			H & H Na/K daily x 2
			Daily PT
			Ancef 1 gm IVPB q 8° x 6 doses
			Coumadin 5 mg PO today
			Call for daily coumadin order
			MS 2-10 mg IM q 4° PRN sev pain
			Percocet 5 mg 1-2 tabs PO q 4° PRN moderate pain
			Compazine 10 mg IM q 6° N/V
			Maalox 15 ml PO PRN
			Dr John Sergen

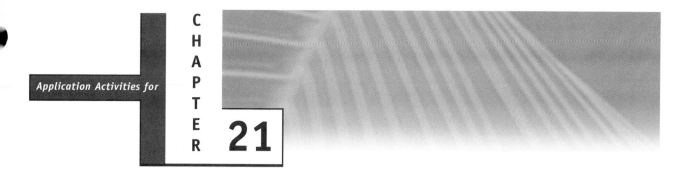

Application Activities for

Recording Vital Signs, Ordering Supplies, Daily Diagnostic Tests, and Filing

Activities in This Chapter

21-1: Record Vital Signs F (Fahrenheit Temperature) and Other Data on a Graphic Record
21-2: Record Vital Signs C (Celsius Temperature) and Other Data on a Graphic Record
21-3: File Records in Patients' Charts (*Optional Activity*)
21-4: Order Daily Diagnostic Tests (*Optional Activity*)

ACTIVITY 21-1

RECORD VITAL SIGNS F (Fahrenheit Temperature) AND OTHER DATA ON A GRAPHIC RECORD

Materials Needed   Black ink pen
Red ink pen (depending on hospital policy)
Labeled graphic record with headings

FIRST DAY

Time	T	P	R	BP	Stool	Wt
0800	100	104	18	136/92	÷	137
1200	100.2®	104	18			
1600	99.8	96	20	120/80	⋰/II	
2000	102	80 a	16			

SECOND DAY

Time	T	P	R	BP	Stool	Wt
0800	98.6 Ⓐ	84	22	120/100	⋅ō	140
1200	97.6	90 a	16			
1600	98	80	18	132/90	⋯/III	
2000	103.2 Ⓡ	60	16			

Figure 21–1

Directions

Practice recording the vital signs and other data shown in the vital signs chart on the graphic record by following the steps below. Refer to the Figure 21–1 for examples. Place a check mark (✓) in the box as you complete each step.

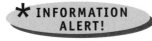

★ INFORMATION ALERT!

Health care facilities and nursing units vary in distribution of responsibilities. Recording vital signs may or may not be the responsibility of the health unit coordinator.

Steps to Record Vital Signs (Fahrenheit Temperature) and Other Data on a Graphic Record

1. Record the Fahrenheit (F) temperature by:
   a. locating the matching temperature in the temperature column on the left side of the graphic record (Fig. 21–2) ❏

4058-3498   6-4-00
3E   Soforth Anne   F- 48
310-1 Dr. U.R.Back

GRAPHIC CHART (Fahrenheit)

Date	6-4-00						6-5-00						6-6-00						6-7-00						6-8-00					
Hospital Days	Admission						1						2						3						4						
Day P.O. or P.P.																															
HOUR	A.M.			P.M.			A.M.			P.M.			A.M.			P.M.			A.M.			P.M.			A.M.			P.M.		
	4	8	12 N	4	8	12 M	4	8	12 N	4	8	12 M	4	8	12 N	4	8	12 M	4	8	12 N	4	8	12 M	4	8	12 N	4	8	12 M

Respirations	18	20	16	22	16	18	16	20	22	22	20																			
Blood Pressure	160/80						130/60																							
Weight																														

	7-3	3-11	11-7	Total	7-3	3-11	11-7	Total	7-3	3-11	11-7	Total	7-3	3-11	11-7	Total	7-3	3-11	11-7	Total
Intake Oral																				
Parenteral																				
Total																				
Output Urine																				
Drainage																				
Emesis																				
Total																				
Stools	i̇	ȯ̇	ȯ̇	ȯ̇	İ	İİ														

00-6000

GRAPHIC CHART (Fahrenheit)

Figure 21–2

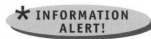

For the first temperature entry, circle the temperature number on the left side of the graphic record. Eventually the record may be microfilmed for storage; this step will indicate which graph line is a temperature.

Example: The Fahrenheit temperature is 100.2°. Circle 100 in the temperature column.

   b. following the correct line to the right (each line is 0.2°) and stopping in the middle of the correct time column under the correct date
   c. placing a solid dot in ink on the line

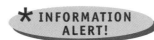

Record an ℝ in ink above the dot to indicate a rectal temperature. Record an Ⓐ in ink above the dot to indicate an axillary temperature. For the first temperature entry, circle the temperature on the left side of the graphic record.

Example: The temperature is 99° in the temperature column. Draw a line to charted temperature. See sample graphic record.

   d. connecting the dot in ink with the previous recorded temperature, if the temperature is not a first entry
   e. drawing a line through the temperature in the vital signs chart to indicate that it has been recorded on the graphic record
2. Record the pulse by
   a. locating the matching pulse in the pulse column on the left side of the graphic record

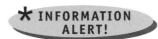

For the first pulse entry, circle the pulse on the left side of the graphic chart.

Example: The pulse is 102. Circle 100 in the pulse column. Draw a line to charted pulse. See sample graphic record.

   b. following the correct line to the right (each line is equal to two counts of a pulse) and stopping in the middle of the correct time column under the appropriate date
   c. placing a solid dot in ink on the line

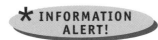

To indicate an apical pulse, record an "a" above the dot.

   d. connecting the dot in ink with the previous recorded pulse, if the pulse is not a first entry
   e. drawing a line through the pulse in the vital signs chart to indicate that it has been recorded on the graphic record
3. Record the respiratory rate by:
   a. locating the respiration heading on the left side of the graphic record
   b. following this row to the right and stopping at the correct time column under the appropriate date

   c. writing the respiratory rate in ink in the space ❏

   d. drawing a line through the respiratory rate in the vital signs chart to indicate that it has been recorded on the graphic record ❏

4. Record the blood pressure by:

   a. locating the blood pressure heading on the left side of the graphic record ❏

   b. following this row to the right and stopping at the correct time column under the appropriate date ❏

   c. writing the blood pressure in ink in the space ❏

   d. drawing a line through the blood pressure in the vital signs chart to indicate that it has been recorded on the graphic record ❏

5. Record the absence or number of stools by:

   a. locating the stool heading on the left side of the graphic chart ❏

   b. following this row to the right and stopping in the correct time column under the appropriate date ❏

   c. writing the symbol for the stools in ink in the space provided on the graphic record ❏

   Example:

   No stools

   One stool

   Two stools

   d. drawing a line through the information on stools in the vital signs chart to indicate that it has been recorded on the graphic chart ❏

6. Record the weight by:

   a. locating the weight column on the left side of the graphic chart ❏

   b. following this row to the right and stopping in the correct time column under the appropriate date ❏

   c. writing the weight in ink in the space ❏

   d. drawing a line through the weight in the vital signs chart to indicate that it has been recorded on the graphic chart ❏

7. Repeat each step as necessary to record the vital signs and other data for each time frame and date. ❏

Place a check mark (✔) in the box below to indicate that you have completed Activity 21–1.

❏ Record Vital Signs F (Fahrenheit Temperature) and Other   Date _____
   Data on the Graphic Chart

➤ **ACTIVITY 21-2**

RECORD VITAL SIGNS C (Celsius Temperature) AND OTHER DATA ON A GRAPHIC RECORD

Materials Needed   Black ink pen

                          Red ink pen (depending on hospital policy)

                          Labeled graphic record with headings

FIRST DAY

Time	P	P	R	BP	Stool	Wt
8:00 A.M.	36.1	82	18	120/80	÷	188
12:00 noon	37	102ᵃ	20			
4:00 P.M.	37.5	98	16			
8:00 P.M.	38.2Ⓡ	80	20	120/80		

Second DAY

Time	T	P	R	BP	Stool	Wt
8:00 A.M.	37.1	88	16	140/100	⊤	190
12:00 noon	34.4	100	20			
4:00 P.M.	36.5	66ᵃ	18			
8:00 P.M.	37Ⓐ	80	22	144/98	⁞‖	

Figure 21–3

Directions

Practice recording the vital signs and other data in shown in vital signs chart (Fig. 21–3) on the graphic record by following the directions and steps in Activity 21–1.

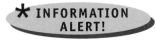
✶ INFORMATION ALERT!

On the Celsius column of the graphic record, each line equals 0.1°.

Place a check mark (✓) in the box below to indicate that you have completed Activity 21–2.

☐ Record Vital Signs C (Celsius Temperature) and Other   Date _____
Data on the Graphic Record

ACTIVITY 21-3

FILE RECORDS IN PATIENTS' CHARTS (Optional Activity)

Materials Needed   Black ink pen
Red ink pen (depending on hospital policy)
Typed records provided by your instructor
Simulated patients' charts provided by your instructor

Situation

It is the end of your shift and several written records (such as diagnostic results and history and physical reports) need to be filed in the patients' charts.

Directions

Practice filing the written reports in the patients' charts using the information in the above situation. Follow the steps below. Place a check mark (✓) in the box as you complete each step.

Steps for Filing Records in Patients' Charts

1. Separate the records according to the patients' names. ❑

2. Check each patient's full name on the chart back with the full name on the record. ❑

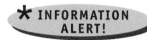

✱ INFORMATION ALERT!

Filing records by room number may result in placing records in the wrong chart. It is important to compare first and last name on the report with the name on chart.

3. Place the record behind the correct chart divider, using consistent sequencing (i.e., reports are filed either to read like a book, or in reverse order with the most recent report first). ❑

Place a check mark (✓) in the box below to indicate that you have completed Activity 21-3.

❑ File Records in Patients' Charts   Date _____

ACTIVITY 21-4

ORDER DAILY DIAGNOSTIC TESTS (Optional Activity)

Materials Needed   Black ink pen

Red ink pen (depending on hospital policy)

Simulated practice Kardex forms provided by your instructor

Diagnostic ordering requisitions

Computer and Practice Activity Software for Transcription of Physicians' Orders

Diagnostic tests: Daily H&H
        Portable chest × 3 days Cl: infiltrates

Dr. Paul Shaffer, D.O.

Directions

Practice ordering the daily diagnostic tests using the simulated Kardex. Follow the steps below. Place a check mark (✓) in the box as you complete each step.

Steps for Ordering Daily Diagnostic Tests

1. Obtain the simulated Kardex. ❑

2. Check each patient's Kardex form for daily diagnostic orders. ❑

3. Order the tests using the computer or complete the corresponding requisition for each daily diagnostic test noted to send to the diagnostic department. ❑

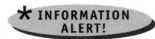

Most hospital computer systems have the capacity to order daily diagnostic tests for days in advance. Daily diagnostic tests should be ordered at a certain time each day (usually 0400 so that the doctor may have the results when making AM rounds) until the doctor discontinues the order.

Place a check mark (✓) in the box below to indicate that you have completed Activity 21–4.

☐ Order Daily Diagnostic Tests   Date _____

Included in Appendix A are sets of doctors' orders that take the patient from admission to discharge or transfer. Many orders are of an advanced nature. They offer the student experience in automatic discontinuation of orders, order changes, and, perhaps most important, orders that have not been presented previously in this manual. The orders are actual sets of doctors' orders obtained from hospitals and are representative of what the student will encounter on the job. If using the Health Unit Coordinator Practice Activity Software for Transcription of Physicians' Orders, choose the patients listed below or admit a new patient (Figure 3) when transcribing each set of orders—the face sheet, lab, and diagnostic imaging reports will match the patient's profile.

Sets of orders include:

Figure A-1 (Parts A through E): 421 ICU—Broderson, Henry: Coronary Artery Bypass Graft (CABG) Surgery
Figure A-2: 404 Med Surg—Garcia, Jose: Post-op Laminectomy

Figure A-3: Admit a new patient: Generalized Pain
Figure A-4: 405-2 Med Surg—Gillium, Patrick: Small Bowel Obstruction
Figure A-5 (Parts A and B): 428-1 Intermediate Care—Monarrez, Joseph: Thoracotomy Surgery
Figure A-6 (Parts A through D): 418 ICU—Parker, Fred: Gastrostomy, Partial Colon Resection, and Colostomy Surgery
Figure A-7 (Parts A and B): 407-1 Med Surg - Jackson, Amy: Laparoscopic Cholecystectomy Surgery

The following orders are handwritten to provide students practice in interpreting doctors' handwriting and medical abbreviations. A typed interpretation of orders, including meaning of medical abbreviations, is included on the back of each set of orders. A typed version will not be available in the hospital, so try to interpret the orders from the handwritten orders prior to looking at the typewritten interpretation.

Admission Orders

PHYSICIANS' ORDER SHEET

DATE	TIME	SYMBOL	ORDERS
0/5/00	1300		Admit to Jcu to Dr. Richters
			Dx: CHF
			Cond: Critical.
			Vitals: Q 2
			ABG on 4L O2
			EKG on ADM; Dx: ARRhythmia
			CXR PA Dx: CHF
			CK MB, trop I stat 798° x 2
			CBC, Cmp, Lytes, Va → today
			Consult Dr. Michaels, cardiothoracic
			surgeon
			Diet: Cardiac
			CBR
			IV: NS c̄ 1/2 DSW @ 8̄cc/HR
			Imdur 60 mg PO q d
			Plavix 75 mg PO q d
			Lopressor 50 mg PO q d
			clonidine 0.1 mg po q 6 hr. —PRN
			if SBP > 180 or DBP > 100
			2D echo Dr. Michaels to read
			Dx: CHF
			Dr. Jack Prunarly MD

Fig. A-1A Coronary artery bypass graft (CABG) surgery orders

— Admit to intensive care unit (ICU) to Dr. Richters
— Diagnosis (Dx): congestive heart failure (CHF)
— Condition: critical
— Vital signs (vitals): every 2 hours (Q 2°)
— Arterial blood gases (ABG) on 4 liters oxygen (4 L O$_2$)
— Electrocardiogram (EKG) on admission (adm); diagnosis (Dx): arrhythmia
— Chest x-Ray (CXR), posteroanterior (PA); diagnosis (DX): congestive heart failure (CHF)
— CKMB, Troponin I stat and every 8 hours times 2 (q 8° × 2)
— Complete blood cell count (CBC), comprehensive metabolic panel (CMP), electrolytes (lytes), urinalysis (Ua) today
— Consult Dr. Michaels, cardiothoracic surgeon
— Diet: cardiac

— Complete bed rest (CBR)
— IV (intravenous) normal saline with ½ 5% dextrose in water (NS c ½ D$_5$W) at (@) 80 cubic centimeteres per hour (80cc/h)
— Imdur 60 milligrams (mg) by mouth (po) every day (qd)
— Plavix 75 milligrams (mg) by mouth (po) every day (qd)
— Lopressor 50 milligrams (mg) by mouth (po)
— clonidine 0.1 milligram (mg) by mouth (po) every 6 hours (q 6°) PRN (as needed) if systolic blood pressure (SBP) greater than (>) 180 or diastolic blood pressure (DBP) greater than (>) 100
— Two-dimension echocardiogram (2 D echo), Dr. Michaels to read; diagnosis (Dx) congestive heart failure (CHF)

Doctor Jack Primary, Medical Doctor

● CKMB: isoenzyme of creatine kinase with muscle and brain subunits, myocardial muscle creatine kinase isoenzyme

Pre-operative Coronary Artery Bypass Graft Orders

PHYSICIANS' ORDER SHEET

DATE	TIME	SYMBOL	ORDERS
05/08	1900		Pre op CABG orders:
			Consent for Coronary Artery Bypass
			graft per Dr. Carl Michaels
			NPO @ 2400
			AM labs: CBC, BMP PT, PTT, Ua
			EKG PRN for Chest pain
			US Vein mapping
			CABG Teaching
			T + X-match 4 U pc, 2 U FPP,
			6 U PLTS
			DC Plavix by 8 pm Tonight
			Tylenol 325 mg II PO q 4° PRN
			pain
			OR by 0630
			Dr. Jacob Primary MD

Fig. A-1B Coronary artery bypass graft (CABG) surgery orders

— Consent for coronary artery bypass graft (CABG) per Dr. Carl Michaels
— Nothing by mouth (NPO) at midnight (@ 2400 hrs)
— AM labs: complete blood cell count (CBC), basic metabolic panel (BMP), prothrombin time (PT), partial thromboplastin time (PTT), urinalysis (UA)
— Electrocardiogram (EKG) as needed (PRN) for chest pain
— Ultrasound (US) vein mapping
— Coronary artery bypass graft (CABG) teaching
— Type and cross (T & X-match) 4 units packed cells (4 U PC), 2 units fresh frozen plasma (2 U FFP), 6 units platelets (6 U Plts)
— Discontinue (DC) Plavix by 8 PM tonight
— Tylenol 325 milligrams (mg) 2 tabs by mouth (po) every 4 hours (q 4°) as needed (PRN) pain
— Operating room (OR) by 0630

Doctor Jack Primary, Medical Doctor

Post-Op Orders

PHYSICIANS' ORDER SHEET

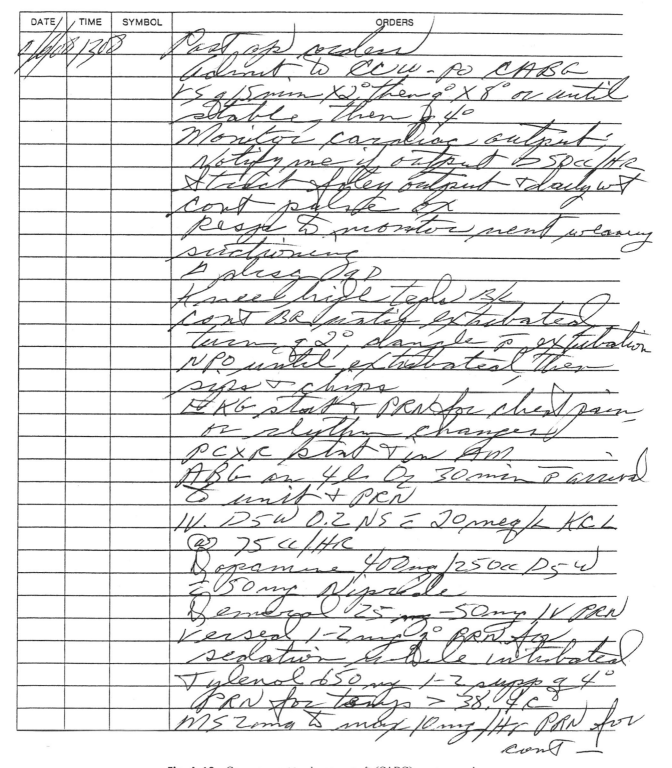

Fig. A-1C Coronary artery bypass graft (CABG) surgery orders

— Admit to coronary care unit (CCU) post op coronary artcry bypass graft (PO CABG)
— Vital signs every 15 minutes times 2 hours (VS q 15 min × 2°), then every hour times eight hours (q° × 8°) or until stable, then every four hours (q 4°)
— Monitor cardiac output; notify me if output is greater than 50 cubic centimeters per hour (> 50 cc per hour)
— Strict foley output and daily weight (wt)
— Continuous pulse oximeter (cont pulse ox)
— Respiratory (resp) to monitor vent weaning, suctioning
— Change dressing every day (Δ drsg qd)
— Knee high teds B/L (bilateral)
— Continuous bedrest (cont BR) unttil extubated, turn every 2 hours (q2°), dangle after (p̄) extubation
— Nothing by mouth (NPO) until extubated, then sips and chips
— Electrocardiogram (EKG) stat and as needed (PRN) for chest pain, or rhythm changes
— Portable chest x-ray (PCXR) stat and in ᴀᴍ
— Arterial blood gases (ABG) on 4 liters oxygen (4L O$_2$) 30 minutes after (p̄) arrival to unit and as needed (PRN)
— Intravenous (IV) 5% dextrose in water and 0.2 normal saline with 20 milliequivalent per liter of potassium chloride at 75 cubic centimeters per hour (D$_5$W 0.2 NS c̄ 20 meq/L KCL at 75cc/hr)
— Dopamine 400 milligrams per 250 cubic centimeters (400 mg/250cc) in 5% dextrose in water (D$_5$W) with (c̄) 50 milligrams (50 mg) Nipride
— Demerol 25 to 50 milligrams (25–50 mg) intravenous as needed (IV prn)
— Versed 1 to 2 milligrams (1–2 mg) every hour (q°) intravenous (IV) as needed (PRN) for sedation while intubated
— Tylenol 650 milligrams (650 mg) 1 to 2 suppositories (1–2 supp) every 4 hours as needed (q 4° PRN) for temperature greater than (temp >) 38.4°C
— Morphine Sulfate (MS) 2 milligrams (2 mg) to maximum 10 milligrams per hour intravenous as needed (max 10mg/h IV PRN) for

Continued on next page

Post-Op Orders—cont'd

PHYSICIANS' ORDER SHEET

Cont —

DATE	TIME	SYMBOL	ORDERS
			prn while intubated
			Compazine 5-10mg IV/IM PRN n/v
			Stat H&H, BMP, CBC, Plts — repeat in AM
			Transfuse 1 u pc for Hct < 60
			PCXR in AM
			EKG in AM
			Dr. Carl Michaels MD

Fig. A-1C (*continued*)   Coronary artery bypass graft (CABG) surgery orders

pain while intubated
— Compazine 5 to 10 milligrams intravenous or intramuscular (5–10 mg IV/IM) as needed for nausea and vomiting (PRN for N/V)
— Stat hemoglobin and hematocrit (H/H), basic metabolic panel (BMP), complete blood cell count (CBC), platelets (plts) — repeat in AM

— Transfuse 1 unit packed cells (1 u PC) for HGB (hemoglobin) less than 60 (<60)
— Portable chest x-ray (PCXR) in AM
— Electrocardiogram (EKG) in AM

Doctor Carl Michael, Medical Doctor

PHYSICIANS' ORDER SHEET

DATE	TIME	SYMBOL	ORDERS
0/7/00	0800		CBC, CMP, PT, PTT, CKMB, H&H in AM.
			PCXR in am DX: Pneumothorax
			OK TO extubate
			ABG in 2 L O2 30 min p̄ extubation
			Morphine 6 – 8 mg PRN for pain post extubation
			C/ flagas tol
			Dr. Jack Primary, MD
0/7/00	0830		DC Dopamine
			DC Demerol
			Dr. Carl Michaels, MD
0/7/00	0730		CBC, CMP, H&H, Plts in AM Va
			PCXR in AM DX: Pneumothorax
			DC Morphine
			Demerol 50 mg Im q 4° pain
			EKG PRN for dysarythmia
			OK To transfer to tele
			Case manager to see regarding placement
			inc diet to full liq
			Dr. Jack Primary, MD

Fig. A-1D Coronary artery bypass graft (CABG) surgery orders

— Complete blood cell count (CBC), comprehensive metabolic panel (CMP), prothrombin time (PT), partial prothrombin plastin time (PTT), CKMB, hemoglobin and hematocrit (H/H) in AM
— Portable chest x-ray (PCXR) in AM; diagnosis (Dx): pneumothorax
— Okay to extubate
— Arterial blood gases (ABG) on 2 liters oxygen (2L O$_2$) 30 minutes after extubation
— Morphine 6 to 8 milligrams (mg) as needed (PRN) for pain post extubation
— Clear liquids as tolerated (cl liq as tol)

Doctor Jack Primary, Medical Doctor

— Discontinue (DC) dopamine
— Discontinue (DC) demerol

Doctor Carl Michaels, Medical Doctor

— Complete blood cell count (CBC), comprehensive metabolic panel (CMP), hemoglobin and hematocrit (H/H), platelets (plts) in AM
— Urinalysis (Ua)
— Portable chest x-ray (PCXR) in am; diagnosis (Dx): pneumothorax
— Discontinue (DC) morphine
— Demerol 50 milligrams (mg) intramuscular (IM) every 4 hours (q 4°) for pain
— Electrocardiogram (EKG) as needed (PRN) for dysrhythmia
— Okay to transfer to telemetry
— Case manager to see regarding placement
— Increase to full liquids (inc diet to full liq)

Doctor Jack Primary, Medical Doctor

PHYSICIANS' ORDER SHEET

DATE	TIME	SYMBOL	ORDERS
0/9/00	0830		CBC CMP in AM
			2 View CXR in AM.
			place transfer orders on chart
			for ē CF
			DC Demerol
			A diet to cardiac
			to Be transferred tomorrow
			Dr. Jacb Runny MD
2/10/00	0900		Transfer to ē CF Today
			send RX c̄ PT
			to see me in 4 wks
			to see Dr. Michaels in 3 wks
			Dr. Jacb Runny MD

Fig. A-1E Coronary artery bypass graft (CABG) surgery orders

— Complete blood cell count (CBC), comprehensive metabolic panel (CMP)
— Two-view chest x-ray (CXR) in AM
— Place transfer orders on chart for extended care facility (ECF)
— Discontinue (DC) demerol
— Change (Δ) diet to cardiac
— To be transferred tomorrow

Doctor Jack Primary, Medical Doctor

— Transfer to extended care facility (ECF) today
— Send prescription (Rx) with (c̄) patient
— To see me in 4 weeks
— To see Dr. Michaels in 3 weeks

Doctor Jack Primary Medical Doctor

Admission Orders

PHYSICIANS' ORDER SHEET

DATE	TIME	SYMBOL	ORDERS
0/5/00	0900		Admit Med Surg - Post-op Lami.
			V.S. Q 4H til STAble, then Q Shift
			Diet mechanical Soft
			up Ad-lib
			I U D5 ½ NS @ 100 cc/Hr D/C when STAble
			LortAb 5mg 1 or 2 po. Q4H PRN PAIN
			Restoril 7.5mg P.O. Q HS PRN Sleep
			DNR STATUS
			Tylenol gr 10 P.O Q 4H PRN
			Resp for SVN Ventolin 2 puff BID
			And PRN
			LOC
			Rehab consult → Dr. Thomas today
			_____ MD
0/6/00	0800		PT/OT Eval → strength training
			TEDS Bil / SCD W/A
			Not Appropriate for Rehab → ECF
			Soc Serv for placement
			_____ MD
0/7/00	0700		D/C to SCF today → PT to follow
			FWW for Ambulation
			_____ MD
0/7/00	0700		CBC, BMP prior to discharge
			_____ MD

Fig. A-2   Post-op laminectomy orders

— Admit to medical surgical post-op laminectomy (Lami)
— Vital signs (VS) every 4 hours until stable (q4 h til stable), then every (Q) shift
— Diet: mechanical soft
— Up as desired (Ad-lib)
— Intravenous (IV) dextrose 5% in ½ normal saline (D_5 ½ NS) at 100 cubic centimeters per hour (100cc/h); Discontinue (D/C) when stable
— Lortab 5 milligrams (mg) 1 or 2 by mouth (po) every 4 hours (q 4 h) as needed (PRN) for pain
— Restoril 7.5 milligrams (mg) by mouth (po) every hour of sleep (Q HS) as needed (PRN) for sleep
— Do not resuscitate (DNR) status
— Tylenol grain (gr) 10 by mouth (po) every 4 hours (Q 4h) as needed (PRN)
— Respiratory (resp) for small volume nebulizer (SVN) Ventolin 2 puffs twice a day (BID) and as needed (PRN)
— Laxative of choice (LOC)
— Rehabilitation (rehab) consult: Doctor Thomas today
　　　　　　　Doctor Melvin Cohen, Medical Doctor

— Physical therapy/occupational therapy (PT/OT) evaluation (eval) for strength training
— Teds bilaterally (Bil) and sequential compression device (SCD) while awake (W/A)
— Not appropriate for rehabilitation (rehab), send to (→) extended care facility (ECF)
— Social services (soc serv) for placement
　　　　　　　Doctor Melvin Cohen, Medical Doctor

— Discharge (D/C) to extended care facility (ECF) today; physical therapy (PT) to follow
— Front-wheeled walker (FWW) for ambulation
　　　　　　　Doctor Melvin Cohen, Medical Doctor

— Complete blood cell count (CBC), basic metabolic panel (BMP) prior to discharge (disch)
　　　　　　　Doctor Melvin Cohen, Medical Doctor

Admission Orders

PHYSICIANS' ORDER SHEET

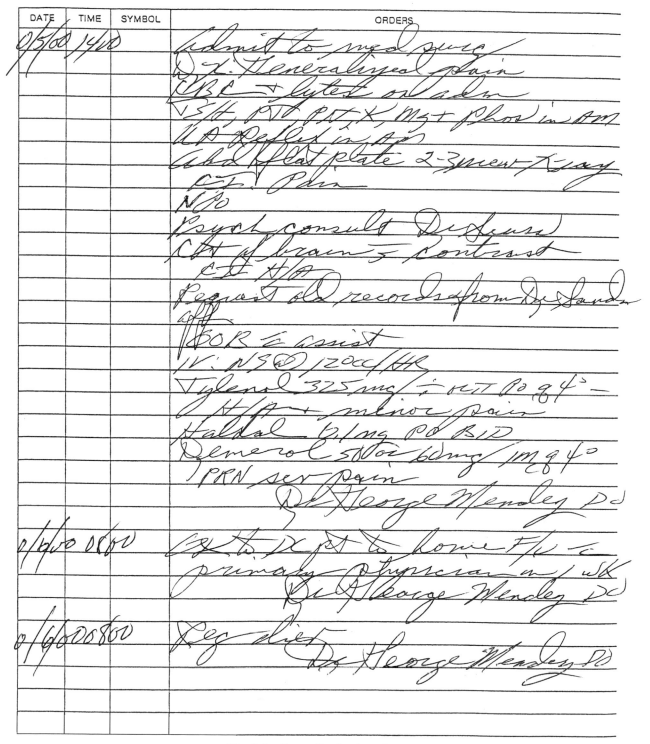

Fig. A-3   Generalized pain orders

— Admit to medical surgical (med surg)
— Diagnosis (Dx): generalized pain
— Complete blood cell count (CBC) and electrolytes (lytes) on admission (adm)
— Thyroid-stimulating hormone (TSH), prothrombin time (PT), partial thromboplastin time (PTT), potassium (K), magnesium (Mg+), phosphorus (Phos) in AM
— Urinalysis (Ua) reflex in AM
— Abdominal (abd) flat plate 2-3 view x-ray; clinical indication (CI): pain
— Nothing by mouth (NPO)
— Psychology (Psych) consult Dr. Seuss
— Computed tomography (CT) of brain without (s̄) contrast clinical indication (CI) headache (H/A)
— Request old records (rec) from Dr. Sand's office (off)
— Out Of Bed (OOB) with (c̄) assistance (assist)
— Intravenous (I.V.) normal saline (NS) at 120 cubic centimeters per hour (cc/h)

— Tylenol 325 milligrams (mg) i or ii by mouth (po) every 4 hours (q 4°) headache (H/A) and minor pain
— Haldol 0.11 milligram (mg) by mouth (po) twice a day (BID)
— Demerol 50–60 milligrams (mg) intramuscular (IM) every 4 hours (q 4°) as needed (PRN) severe (sev) pain
   Doctor George Mendez, Doctor of Osteopathy

— Ok to discharge patient to home; follow up (F/U) with (c̄) primary physician in 1 week (wk)
   Doctor George Mendez, Doctor of Osteopathy

— Regular diet
   Doctor George Mendez, Doctor of Osteopathy

Admission Orders

PHYSICIANS' ORDER SHEET

DATE	TIME	SYMBOL	ORDERS
00/0/00/300			ADMIT TO 2A
			DX: SMALL BOWEL OBSTRUCTION
			NPO
			CONSULT DR SMITH – GASTRO
			ABD CT CI: SMALL BOWEL OBSTRUK
			CBC BMP on ADM
			UA
			EKG CI: ARRHYTHMIA
			REQUEST OLD RECORDS
			ABD X RAY FILMS TO FLOOR
			CONSENT FOR EGD – PSS BX SCHED FOR AM
			TWE DR CL
			POST EGD: CL UD W/O
			Dr Philip Lewis MD
00/07/00/330			PERCOCET 325 mg PO PRN FOR PAIN
			TYLENOL 325 mg PO PRN H/A – MINOR PAIN
			Dr Philip Lewis MD
0/8/00 0800			OK TO DC TODAY
			RESUME ALL HOME MEDS
			MAY SHOWER
			F/U IN MY OFFICE IN 1 WK
			Dr Philip Lewis MD

Fig. A-4 Small bowel obstruction orders

— Admit to 2A
— Diagnosis (Dx): small bowel obstruction
— Nothing by mouth (NPO)
— Consult Dr. Smith, Gastroenterology (Gastro)
— Abdominal computed tomography (abd CT), Clinical indication (CI) small bowel obstruction (obstruc)
— Complete blood cell count (CBC)—basic metabolic panel (BMP) on admission (adm)
— Urinalysis (Ua)
— Electrocardiogram (EKG) clinical indication: arrhythmia
— Request old records
— Abdominal (abd) x-ray films to floor
— Consent for esophagogastroduodenoscopy (EGD)—possible biopsy (poss Bx) scheduled (sched) for AM
— Tap water enemas (TWE) until clear (til cl)

— Post esophagogastroduodenoscopy (EGD): clear liquids when awake (cl liq W/A)
Doctor Philip Lewis, Medical Doctor

— Percocet 325 milligrams (mg) by mouth (po) as needed (PRN) for pain
— Tylenol 325 milligrams (mg) by mouth (po) as needed (PRN) headache (H/A)—minor pain
Doctor Philip Lewis, Medical Doctor

— Okay to discharge (D/C) today
— Resume all home medications (meds)
— May shower
— Follow up (F/U) in my office in 1 week (wk)
Doctor Philip Lewis, Medical Doctor

Pre-Op Thoracotomy Orders

PHYSICIANS' ORDER SHEET

DATE	TIME	SYMBOL	ORDERS
1/7/00	0900		Pre-op Thoracotomy Ord. Permit for Thoracotomy, Chest tube placement, Possible Removal of lesions. NPO p MN s for meds. Vancomycin 1 g IV ā 12° Pneumatic hose Rt LE. Synthroid 0.2 mg PO D5W ½ NS TKO. Vancomycin Peak & Trough around 3rd dose. _Susan Balshaw MD_
1/8/00	1300		D/C U/C by pts for surg. _Dr. Susan Balshaw_
1/8/00	1430		Demerol 100 mg ⎫ Vistaril 25 mg ⎬ im on call to OR Restoril 15 mg PO HS. _Dr. Thomas Whitfield MD_

Fig. A-5A Thoracotomy surgery orders

— Permit for thoracotomy with (c̄) chest tube placement, possible biopsy (bx), removal of lesions
— Nothing by mouth (NPO) after (p̄) midnight (MN) except for (s̄) meds
— vancomycin 1 grain (1g) intravenous (IV) every 12 hours (q 12°)
— Pneumatic hose to operating room (OR)
— No known drug allergies (NKDA)
— Synthroid 0.2 milligram (mg) by mouth (PO) every day (qd)
— Dextrose 5% in water with ½ normal saline (D$_5$W ½ NS) to keep open (TKO)
— vancomycin peak and trough around third dose

           Doctor Susan Balstran, Medical Doctor

— Type and cross-match (T & X) 2 units (2U) packed cells (PC), 6 units (6U) platelets (plts) for surgery (surg)

           Doctor Susan Balstran, Medical Doctor

Demerol 100 milligrams (mg) ⎤ intramuscular (IM) on call
Vistaril 25 milligrams (mg) ⎦ to operating room (OR)
Restoril 15 milligrams (mg) by mouth (PO) hour of sleep (HS)

           Doctor Thomas Whitiker, Medical Doctor

Post-Op Orders

PHYSICIANS' ORDER SHEET

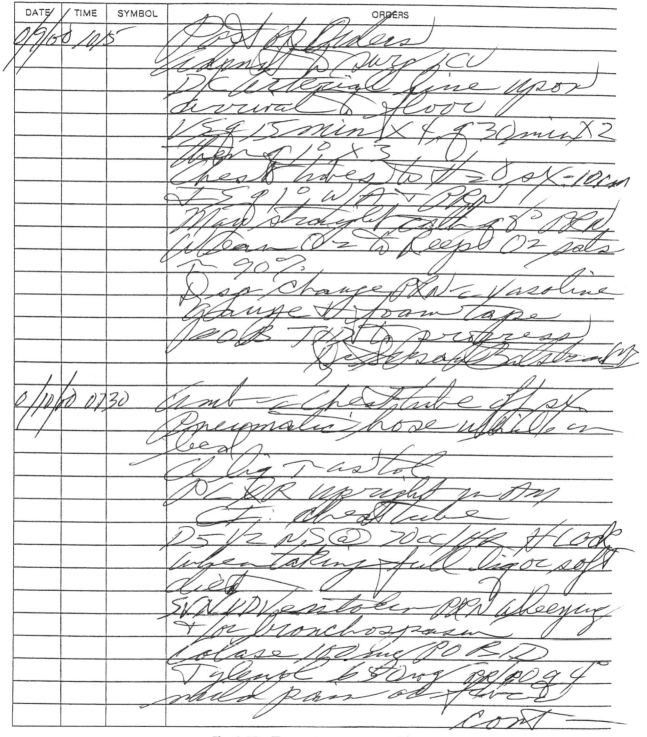

Fig. A-5B Thoracotomy surgery orders

— Admit to surgical intensive care unit (surg ICU)
— Discontinue (Disc) arterial line upon arrival to floor
— Vital signs (VS) every 15 minutes times 4 (q 15 min × 4), every 30 minutes times 2 (q 30 min × 2), then every one hour times 3 (q 1° × 3)
— Chest tubes to water suction (H_2O Sx)—10 centimeters (10 cm)
— Incentive spirometry (IS) every hour (q 1h) while awake (W/A) and when necessary (PRN)
— May straight catheterize (cath) every 8 hours (q 8h) as needed (PRN)
— Wean oxygen (O_2) to keep oxygen saturation (O_2 sats) above 90% (↑ 90%)
— Dressing (drsg) changes as needed (PRN) with (c̄) Vasoline gauze and foam tape
— Out of bed (OOB) three times a day (TID) to progress

Doctor Susan Balstran, Medical Doctor

— Ambulate (amb) with (c̄) chest tube off suction (SX)
— Pneumatic hose while in bed
— Clear liquids advance as tolerated (cl liq ↑ as tol)
— Portable Chest x-ray (PCXR) upright in AM; clinical indication—chest tube
— Dextrose 5% with ½ normal saline (D_5 ½ NS) at 70 cubic centimeters per hour (70 cc/h); heplock when taking full liquids (liq) or soft diet
— Small volume nebulizer (SVN) unit dose (UD) Ventolin as needed (PRN) wheezing and/or bronchospasm
— Colace 100 milligrams (mg) by mouth (PO) twice a day (BID)
— Tylenol 650 milligrams (mg) per rectum or by mouth (PR/PO) every 4 hours (q 4°) as needed (PRN) for mild pain or fever

Continued

Post-Op Orders—cont'd

PHYSICIANS' ORDER SHEET

DATE	TIME	SYMBOL	ORDERS
			Compazine 5-10 mg IV/IM q 6° PRN N/V
			Restoril 7.5 mg PO q HS PRN
			Synthroid 0.2 mg PO qd
			Dr. Susan Bertram MD
0/10/00	1400		CBC
			CMP in AM
			Dr. Susan Bertram MD
0/11/00	0700		DC O₂ chest tube
			Dsg abd drain site q8° PRN
			Clr diet & prog
			Dr. Susan Bertram MD
0/12/00	0710		DC chest tube
			Leave occlusive dsg on chest tube site × 48°
			PA & lat chest in AM & for infiltrates
			Dr. Susan Bertram MD
0/13/00	0800		May DC IV today
			May remove occlusive dsg tomorrow. Shower in 2 days
			Fll csurgeon in 2 wks
			Dr. Susan Bertram MD

Fig. A-5B (*continued*) Thoracotomy surgery orders

— Compazine 5 to 10 milligrams (5–10 mg) intravenous or intramuscular (IV/IM) every 6 hours (q 6h) as needed (PRN) for nausea and vomiting (N/V)
— Restoril 7.5 milligrams (mg) by mouth (PO) every hour of sleep (q HS)
— Bowel care of choice (BCOC)
— Synthroid 0.2 milligram (mg) by mouth (PO) every day (qd)

Doctor Susan Balstran, Medical Doctor

— Complete blood cell count (CBC)
— Comprehensive metabolic panel (CMP) } in AM

Doctor Susan Balstran, Medical Doctor

— Discontinue (DC) suction (Sx) to chest tube
— Change dressing (Δ drsg) abdominal (abd) drain site every day (qd) as needed (PRN)
— Increase (inc) diet to regular (reg)

Doctor Susan Balstran, Medical Doctor

— Discontinue (DC) chest tube
— Leave occlusive dressing (drsg) on chest tube site times 48 hrs (× 48°)
— Posteroanterior and lateral (PA & lat) chest (x-ray) in AM for infiltrates

Doctor Susan Balstran, Medical Doctor

— May discharge (disch) home today
— Discontinue (DC) intravenous (IV)
— May remove occlusive dressing (drsg) tomorrow—shower in 2 days
— Follow up (F/U) with (c̄) surgeon in 2 weeks (wks)

Doctor Susan Balstran, Medical Doctor

Admission Orders

PHYSICIANS' ORDER SHEET

DATE	TIME	SYMBOL	ORDERS
0/8/00	0930		Admit to med Surg
			Dx: Abd Pain + diarrhea
			Full Code Status
			BRP c̄ assist
			NPO
			EKG, CXR PA + LAT upon adm if not done in ED
			IVF: 0.9 NS @ 125cc/h
			Timoptic ophth sol 0.25% 1 gtt OS Bid
			Phenergan 12.5 mg IV q 3h PRN for restlessness
			Demerol 12.5 mg IV q h PRN for pain
			CMP, CBC c̄ diff in AM
			CT of abd/Pelvis c̄ IV + Po contrast now for abd pain
			Valley Surg for consult regarding small bowel obstruction/abd pain
			SVN - albuterol q 8h UD
			Notify MD of any problems
			Dr. ___ Harrington MP
0/9/00	0700		Bld C/ x 2 Stat
			CBC q AM
			Cimetidine 300 mg Po qid: first dose now
			Place Foley to st drainage
			NG to intermittent Sx
			Dr. Pat Harrington MD

Fig. A-6A   Gastrostomy, partial colon resection, and colostomy surgery orders

— Admit to medical surgical (med surg)
— Diagnosis (Dx): abdominal (abd) pain and diarrhea
— Full code status
— Bathroom privileges with assistance (BRP c̄ assist)
— Nothing by mouth (NPO)
— Electrocardiogram (EKG), chest x-ray posteroanterior (CXR PA) and lateral (& lat) upon admission if not done in emergency department (ED)
— Intravenous fluids (IVF): 0.9 normal saline (NS) at 125 cubic centimeters per hour (125 cc/h)
— Timoptic ophthalmic solution (ophth sol) 0.25% 1 drop (gtt) left eye (OS) twice a day (Bid)
— Phenergan 12.5 milligrams (mg) intravenous (IV) every 3 hours (q 3h) as needed (prn) for restlessness
— Demerol 12.5 milligrams (mg) intravenous (IV) every hour (q h) for pain
— Comprehensive metabolic panel (CMP), complete blood cell count with differential (CBC c̄ diff) in AM

— Computed tomography (CT) of abdomen (abd)/pelvis with (c̄) intravenous (IV) and by mouth (PO) contrast now for abdominal (abd) pain
— Valley Surgical (Surg) for consult regarding small bowel obstruction/abdominal (abd) pain
— Small volume nebulizer (SVN) – Albuterol every 8 hours (q 8h) unit dose (UD)
— Notify medical doctor (MD) of any problems
Doctor Pat Harrington, Medical Doctor

— Blood culture (Bld Cx) times 2 (× 2) stat
— Complete blood cell count (CBC) every AM (q am)
— Cimetidine 300 milligram (mg) by mouth (po) four times a day (qid)—first dose now
— Place Foley catheter (cath) to straight (st) drainage
— Nasogastric (NG) to intermittent suction (Sx)
Doctor Pat Harrington, Medical Doctor

Pre-Op Orders

PHYSICIANS' ORDER SHEET

DATE	TIME	SYMBOL	ORDERS
0/9/00	1310		Pre-Op Orders:
			Keep NPO
			Surg consent for gastrostomy c̄ partial
			colon resection + colostomy
			T + X match 2 u PC for Surg 0700
			Add 20 meq KCL to IVF
			SCD while in bed
			Disc cimitidine
			Pepcid 20 mg IV Bid
			Valley Anesthesia for pre op orders
			Dr. Pat Farrington MD
0/9/00	1500		NPO 2400
			Demerol 125 mg ⎫
			Vistaril 25 mg ⎬ IM on call to OR
			Restoril 30 mg HS MR X1
			Dr Joanne Torres MD

Fig. A-6B Gastrostomy, partial colon resection, and colostomy surgery orders

— Keep nothing by mouth (NPO)
— Surgical (Surg) consent for gastrostomy with (c̄) partial colon resection and colostomy
— Type and crossmatch (T & X-match) 2 units (2 U) packed cells (PC) for surgery (surg) 0700
— Add 20 milliequivalent (mEq) potassium chloride (KCl) to intravenous fluids (IVF)
— Sequential compression device (SCD) while in bed
— Discontinue (Disc) cimetidine
— Pepcid 20 milligram (mg) intravenous (IV) twice a day (bid)
— Valley anesthesia for pre-op orders

Doctor Pat Harrington, Medical Doctor

— Nothing by mouth (NPO) midnight (2400)
— Demerol 125 milligrams (mg) } Intramuscular (IM)
— Vistaril 25 milligrams (mg) } on call to operating room (OR)
— Restoril 30 milligrams (mg) per hour of sleep (HS) may repeat time 1 (MR × 1)

Doctor Joanne Torres, Medical Doctor

Post Op Orders

PHYSICIANS' ORDER SHEET

DATE	TIME	SYMBOL	ORDERS
9/10/00	1215		Post-op orders:
			Admit to Surg ICU
			VS per PO root
			Strict I + O q shift
			↑ HOB 30°
			IS q 4h
			NG to lo intermittent Sx
			Foley to St drain
			O₂ to keep sats ↑ 90%
			SCD
			Demerol 50 mg IV q 4h pain
			Vistaril 25 mg IM q 6h for N/V
			Cipro 200 mg IV q 12h
			Lovenox 30 mg sq Bid
			Daily CBC, PH+ Ct, PH, PH
			PCXR in AM cf infiltrates
			R. A. Harrington MD
9/11/00	1000		Consult infectious disease
			hydrocortisone 100 mg IV q 12h
			BVN Ventolyn q 6h UD
			Sump drains to cont Sx
			Cl liq as tol
			R. Pat Harrington MD

Fig. A-6C   Gastrostomy, partial colon resection, and colostomy surgery orders

— Admit to surgical intensive care unit (Surg ICU)
— Vital signs (VS) per post-op routine (post-op rout)
— Strict intake and output (I & O) every (q) shift
— Elevate head of bed 30° (↑ HOB 30 degrees)
— Incentive spirometry (IS) every 4 hours (q 4 h)
— Nasal gastric (NG) to low (lo) intermittent suction (Sx)
— Foley to straight (st) drain
— Oxygen (O$_2$) to keep saturation (sats) above 90% (↑ 90%)
— Sequential compression device (SCD)
— Demerol 50 milligrams (mg) intravenous (IV) every 4 hours (q 4h) pain
— Vistaril 25 milligrams (mg) intramuscular (IM) every 4 hours (q 6h) for nausea and vomiting (N/V)
— Cipro 200 milligrams (mg) intravenous (IV) every 12 hours (q 12h)

— Lovenox 30 milligrams (mg) subcutaneous (sq) twice a day (Bid)
— Daily complete blood cell count (CBC), platelet count (Plt Ct), prothrombin time (PT), partial thromboplastin time (PTT)
— Portable chest x-ray (PCXR) in AM; clinical indication (CI): infiltrates

Doctor Pat Harrington, Medical Doctor

Consult infectious disease
hydrocortisone 100 milligrams (mg) intravenous (IV) every 12 hours (q 12h)
Small-volume nebulizer (SVN) every 6 hours (q 6h) unit dose (UD)
Sump drain to continuous (cont) suction (Sx)
Clear liquids as tolerated (Cl liq as tol)

Doctor Pat Harrington, Medical Doctor

PHYSICIANS' ORDER SHEET

DATE	TIME	SYMBOL	ORDERS
9/12/00	0940		Trans to floor unit
			If fever > 100°, notify Infec disease
			Disc Foley
			Amb as tol
			Adv DAT
			Disc Demerol
			Disc NG Sx
			Disc SCD
			Case mgt to arrange home IV antibiotic therapy
			Ostomy nurse to see pt for colostomy care
			Dr. Pat Harrington MD
9/13/00	0730		OK to disch home today
			Fax disch ord to Infectious disease + my office
			F/U in my office in 10 days
			Dr. Pat Harrington MD

Fig. A-6D   Gastrostomy, partial colon resection, and colostomy surgery orders

— Transfer (Trans) to floor unit
— If fever greater than (>) 100°, notify Infectious (infec) Disease
— Discontinue (Disc) Foley
— Ambulate as tolerated (Amb as tol)
— Advance diet as tolerated (Adv DAT)
— Discontinue (Disc) Demerol
— Discontinue (Disc) nasal gastric suction (NG Sx)
— Discontinue (Disc) sequential compression device (SCD)

— Case management (mgt) to arrange home intravenous (IV) antibiotic therapy
— Ostomy nurse to see patient (pt) for colostomy care

Doctor Pat Harrington, Medical Doctor

— OK to discharge (disch) home today
— Fax discharge (disch) orders (ord) to Infectious Disease and my office
— Follow up (F/U) in my office in 10 days

Doctor Pat Harrington, Medical Doctor

Admission Orders

PHYSICIANS' ORDER SHEET

DATE	TIME	SYMBOL	ORDERS
0/9/00	0920		Admit to med/surg unit
			DX: Cholecystitis
			Consult - Dr. John Payton
			NPO
			I.V.: NS 60 cc /hr Call if infiltates
			MS 4 mg IV q 4° PRN pain
			consent for Laparoscopic
			Cholecystectomy
			on call to OR @ 0700
			T + X 2 u PRBC
			CBC + CMP in A.M. Results on chart
			Dr. Paul Taylor MD
0/9/00	1400		DC MS
			Tylenol 325 mg PO 1-2 tab q 4° pain
			Dr. Paul Taylor MD
0/9/00	1920		Demerol 125 mg ⎫ IM
			Phenergan 25 mg ⎭ 0700
			Ambien 15 mg PO HS may repeat X 1
			Dr. John Peters MD

Fig. A-7A Laparoscopic cholecystectomy surgery orders

— Admit to medical/surgical (med/surg) unit
— Diagnosis (Dx): cholecystitis
— Consult Dr. John Payton
— Nothing by mouth (NPO)
— Intravenous (IV) normal saline (NS) 60 cubic centimeters per hour (cc/h)
— Morphine sulfate (MS) 4 milligrams 4 (mg) intravenous (IV) every 4 hours (q 4°) as needed (prn) pain
— Consent for laparoscopic cholecystectomy
— On call to operating room (OR) at 0700
— Type and Cross (T & X) 2 units (u) packed red blood cells (PRBC)
— Complete blood cell count (CBC) and comprehensive metabolic panel (CMP) in AM. Results on chart

Doctor Paul Taylor Medical Doctor

— Discontinue (DC) morphine sulfate (MS)
— Tylenol 325 milligrams (mg) by mouth (PO) 1–2 tab every 4 hours (q 4°) pain

Doctor Paul Taylor, Medical Doctor

— Demerol 125 milligrams (mg) ⎤ intramuscular (IM)
— Phenergan 25 milligrams (mg) ⎦ 0700
— Ambien 15 milligrams (mg) by mouth (PO) hour of sleep (HS) may repeat times (×) 1

Doctor John Peters, Medical Doctor

Post-Op Orders

PHYSICIANS' ORDER SHEET

DATE	TIME	SYMBOL	ORDERS
9/10/00	1100		Post-op orders
			Rout. Pl. VS
			Strict I + O
			↑ HOB 30°
			OOB c̄ assist
			Start cl liq adv DAT
			No ice-straws
			IV: D5NS c̄ 20 mEq K @ .75cc/hr til
			no N/V, then hep lock
			Cipro 250mg PO q 12°
			Ambien 5 mg PO HS
			Compazine 10 mg IM q 6° PRN for N/V
			MSO4 4-6 mg IM q 4° PRN for sev pain
			Percocet 5mg 1-2 tabs PO q 4° mild pain
			H + H in A.M.
			PT + OT to eval + treat
			Dr. Paul Taylor MD
9/11/00	0645		DC MS
			DC Compazine
			inc. diet to reg - lactose restrict
			CBC + SMP this A.M.
			SS consult for home health IV
			antibiotics
			Dr. Paul Taylor MD
9/12/00	1800		D/C to home P̄ PA + lat CXR
			F/U in my office in 1 wk
			Dr. Paul Taylor MD

Fig. A-7B Laparoscopic cholecystectomy surgery orders

— Routine post-op (P.O.) vital signs (VS)
— Strict intake and output (I and O)
— Elevate (↑) Head of Bed 30 degrees (HOB 30°)
— Out of bed (OOB) with assist (c̄ assist)
— Start clear liquids (cl liq), advance diet as tolerated (adv DAT)
— No ice—straws
— Intravenous (IV): dextrose 5% in normal saline (D_5NS) with 20 milliequivalent potassium (20 mEq K) at 75 cubic centimeters per hour (cc/h) until no nausea and vomiting (til no N/V), then heplock
— Cipro 250 milligrams (mg) by mouth (PO) every 12 hours (q12°)
— Ambien 15 milligrams (mg) by mouth at hour of sleep (PO HS)
— Compazine 10 milligrams (mg) intramuscular (IM) every 6 hours (q 6°) per rectum (PR) for nausea/vomiting (N/V)
— Morphine sulfate (MS) 4–6 mg intramuscular (IM) every 4 hours (q 4°) as needed (PRN) for Severe (sev) pain

— Percocet 5 milligram (mg) 1–2 tablets (tabs) by mouth (PO) every 4 hours (q 4°) mild pain
— Hemoglobin and hematocrit (H & H) in AM
— Physical therapy (PT) and occupational therapy (OT) to evaluate (eval) and treat

        Doctor Paul Taylor, Medical Doctor

— Discontinue (DC) morphine sulfate (MS)
— Discontinue (DC) compazine
— Increase (inc) diet to regular (reg), lactose restrict
— Complete blood cell count (CBC) and basic metabolic panel (BMP) in AM
— Social services (SS) consult for home health intravenous (IV) antibiotics

        Doctor Paul Taylor, Medical Doctor

— Discharge (D/C) to home after (p̄) posteroanterior and lateral (PA & lat) chest x-ray (CXR)
— Follow up (F/U) in my office in 1 week (wk)

        Doctor Paul Taylor, Medical Doctor

Generic Hospital Forms and Examples of Computer Screens That May Be Used as Ordering Requisitions When Computers Are Not Available

These hospital forms and examples of computer screens are designed to match the activities included in the Manual. For use by students in the classroom setting, remove the forms and reproduce as many as are needed to complete the activities.

The examples of computer screens may be used as requisitions for ordering supplies, tests, and procedures. A CD-ROM titled: *Practice Activity Software for Transcription of Physicians' Orders* packaged with this Manual is for use in place of the requisitions when a computer is available. Patient chart forms, including admission packet forms, surgery consent form, graphic form, and blood transfusion consent forms, are available on the CD and may be printed as needed.

PATIENT ACTIVITY SHEET

Room Number	Patient's Name	Activity

ADMISSION AGREEMENT (CONDITION OF ADMISSION)

Patient or someone acting for the patient agrees to the following terms of hospital admission.

1) **MEDICAL TREATMENT:** Patient will be treated by his/her attending doctor or specialists. Patient authorizes Hospital to perform services ordered by the doctors. Special consent forms may be needed. Many doctors and assistants (such as those providing x-rays, lab tests, and anesthesiology) may not be Hospital employees and are responsible for their own treatment activities.

2) **GENERAL DUTY NURSING:** Hospital provides only general nursing care. If the patient needs special or private nursing, it must be arranged by the patient or by the doctor treating the patient.

3) **MONEY AND VALUABLES:** The Hospital has a safe in which to keep money or valuables. It will not be responsible for any loss or damage to items not deposited in the safe. The Hospital will not be responsible for loss or damage to items such as glasses, dentures, hearing aids and contact lenses.

4) **TEACHING PROGRAMS:** The Hospital participates in programs for training of health care personnel. Some services may be provided to the patient by persons in training under the supervision and instruction of doctors or hospital employees. These persons may also observe care given to the patient by doctors and hospital employees. Photos or video tapes may be made of surgical procedures.

5) **RELEASE OF INFORMATION:** The Hospital may disclose all or any part of the patient's medical and/or financial records (INCLUDING INFORMATION REGARDING ALCOHOL OR DRUG ABUSE), to the following:

   a. **Third Party Payors:** Any person or corporation, or their designee, which is or may be liable under a contract to the hospital, the patient, a family member, or employer of the patient, for payment of all or part of the hospital's charges, including but not limited to, insurance companies, utilization review organizations, workman's compensation payors, hospital or medical service companies, welfare funds, governmental agencies or the patient's employer;

   b. **Medical Audit:** The Hospital conducts a program of medical audit and the patient's medical information may be reviewed and released by employees, members of the medical staff or other authorized persons to appropriate agencies as part of this program.

   c. **Medical Research:** Information may be released for use in medical studies and medical research.

   d. **Other Health Care Providers:** Information may be released to other health care providers in order to provide continued patient care.

   I understand that the authorization granted in items 5. a, b, c and d may be revoked by me at any time, except to the extent to which action has been taken in reliance upon it. The authorization will stay in effect as long as the need for information in items 5. a, b, c and d exist.

I have read and understand this Admissions Agreement, have received a copy and I am the patient, the parent of a minor child or the court appointed guardian for the patient and am authorized to act on the patient's behalf to sign this Agreement.

_____   _____
WITNESS   PATIENT   PARENT OF MINOR CHILD   COURT APPOINTED GUARDIAN
                                                                             (PLEASE CIRCLE THE CORRECT TITLE)

_____
DATE   TIME

MEDICAL POWER OF ATTORNEY A.R.S. §14-5501: I appoint_____

_____   _____
ADDRESS   PHONE
as my agent to act in all matters relating to my health care, including full power to give or refuse consent to all medical, surgical and hospital care. This power of attorney shall be effective upon my disability or incapacity or when there is uncertainty whether I am dead or alive and shall have the same effect as if I were alive, competent, and able to act for myself.

_____   _____
WITNESS   PATIENT

FINANCIAL AGREEMENT

I agree that in return for the services provided to the patient, I will pay the account of the patient, and/or prior to discharge make financial arrangements satisfactory to the hospital for payment. If the account is sent to an attorney for collection, I agree to pay reasonable attorney's fees and collection expenses. The amount of the attorney's fee shall be established by the Court and not by a Jury in any court action. A delinquent account may be charged interest at the legal rate.

If any signer is entitled to hospital benefits of any type whatsoever under any policy of insurance insuring patient, or any other party liable to patient, the benefits are hereby assigned to hospital for application on patient's bill. However, IT IS UNDERSTOOD THAT THE UNDERSIGNED AND PATIENT ARE PRIMARILY RESPONSIBLE FOR PAYMENT OF PATIENT'S BILL.

IN GRANTING ADMISSION OR RENDERING TREATMENT, THE HOSPITAL IS RELYING ON MY AGREEMENT TO PAY THE ACCOUNT. EMERGENCY CARE WILL BE PROVIDED WITHOUT REGARD TO THE ABILITY TO PAY.

_____   _____
PATIENT   OTHER PARTY AGREEING TO PAY

_____   _____
WITNESS   RELATIONSHIP TO PATIENT

_____
DATE

PATIENT PROFILE (FACE SHEET)

1 PATIENT HOSP.NO.(M.R.#)	INFO STATUS		ACCOUNT NO. (BUS. OFF.)

PATIENT NAME	LAST	FIRST	MIDDLE	ADM. DATE MO. / DAY / YR.	ADM. TIME	HOW BROUGHT TO HOSPITAL
2						

PATIENT'S CURRENT ADDRESS	STREET, P.O. BOX, APT. NO.	CITY	STATE	ZIP CODE	TELEPHONE NO.
3					

PATIENT'S PERMANENT ADDRESS	STREET, P.O. BOX, APT. NO.	CITY	STATE	ZIP CODE	TELEPHONE NO.
4					

SEX 1. MALE 2. FEMALE	MARITAL STATUS 1. SINGLE 4. DIVORCED 2. MARRIED 5. WIDOWED 3. SEPARATED	RACE 1. WHITE 4. ORIENTAL 2. BLACK 5. OTHER 3. INDIAN	RELIGION 3. PROTESTANT 1. CATHOLIC 4. OTHER 2. JEWISH 5. LDS	AREA OF RESIDENCE
5				

BIRTHDATE	AGE	PLACE OF BIRTH	MAIDEN NAME	SOC. SEC. NO./MEDICARE NO.
6				

PATIENT'S OCCUPATION	UNION & LOCAL NO.	PATIENT'S EMPLOYER	ADDRESS	TELEPHONE NO.
7				

PREVIOUSLY TREATED HERE? ☐ YES NAME ☐ NO USED	PREV. ADM. DATE	MO. DA. YR.	PREV. ADMISSION 1. INPATIENT 2. OUTPATIENT	IF NEWBORN, MOTHER'S HOSP. NO.
8				

UNIT	ROOM NO.	ACCOM. CODES	1. PRI 3. NURSERY 5. ICU 7. CCU 2. SEMI 4. PREMIE 6. RCU 8. VIP	ROOM RATE	PAY STATUS	CLASS OF ADMISSION 1. EMERGENCY 3. URGENT 2. ELECTIVE 4. OTHER
9						

ADMITTING DIAGNOSIS
10

PHYSICIAN NAME	PHYSICIAN NO.	ADM. SERVICE	INFORMATION OBTAINED FROM:
11			

SPOUSE OR NEAREST RELATIVE (NEXT OF KIN)	RELATIONSHIP	ADDRESS	TELEPHONE NO.
12			

SECOND RELATIVE OR FRIEND	RELATIONSHIP	ADDRESS	TELEPHONE NO.
13			

RESPONSIBLE PARTY NAME	RELATIONSHIP	SOC. SEC. NO.
14		

RESP. PARTY ADDRESS	STREET P.O. BOX APT. NO.	CITY	STATE	ZIP CODE	TELEPHONE NO.
15					

RESP. PARTY OCCUPATION	NO. YRS. IN THIS EMPLOY	RESP. PARTY EMPLOYER	ADDRESS	TELEPHONE NO.
16				

LENGTH OF TIME IN ARIZ.	1. OWN HOME 2. RENT HOME	TYPE OF HOME	BANK NAME & BRANCH	1. SAVINGS 2. CHECKING
17				

CREDIT REFERENCES	1. NAME	ADDRESS	TELEPHONE NO.
18			
19	2. NAME	ADDRESS	TELEPHONE NO.

INDUSTRIAL INJURY	DATE:	MO. DA. YR.	CLAIM NO.	EMPLOYER'S NAME AND ADDRESS AT TIME OF INJURY
20				

BLUE CROSS	NAME OF PLAN	GROUP NO.	IDENTIFICATION	EFFECTIVE DATE MO. DA. YR.	CITY	STATE
21						

CHAMPUS DATA	PATIENT'S ID NO.	CARD EFFECTIVE MO. DA. YR.	CARD EXPIRES ON MO. DA. YR.	PATIENT OR SPONSORS BRANCH OF SERVICE	SERVICE CARD NO.
22					
23	SPONSORS NAME	RANK-SERVICE NO.	DUTY STATION		

OTHER INSURANCE (INC. BLOOD BANK & BLUE SHIELD)	INS. CO. NO.	COMPANY NAME	POLICY HOLDER NAME	POLICY NO.	DATE ISSUED MO. DA. YR.	CITY	STATE
24							
25	INS. CO. NO.	COMPANY NAME	POLICY HOLDER NAME	POLICY NO.	DATE ISSUED MO. DA. YR.	CITY	STATE

NAME OF HEALTH FACILITY DISCHARGED FROM WITHIN LAST 60 DAYS	ADDRESS
26	

OTHER INFO.	V. A. ☐	COORDINATION OF BENEFITS ☐	INTERVIEWED BY	TYPED BY
27				

28 REMARKS:

	PHYSICIANS' ORDER SHEET		

DATE	TIME	SYMBOL	ORDERS

GRAPHIC CHART

Date																										
Hospital Days																										
Day P.O. or P.P.																										
HOUR		A.M.			P.M.			A.M.			P.M.			A.M.			P.M.			A.M.			P.M.			
		4	8	12 N	4	8	12 M	4	8	12 N	4	8	12 M	4	8	12 N	4	8	12 M	4	8	12 N	4	8	12 M	

PULSE (Red) — **TEMPERATURE (Black)** — **RECTAL / ORAL**

F	C
150	106° 41°
	105°
140	104° 40°
130	103°
120	102° 39°
110	101°
100	100° 38°
90	99°
80	98.6° 37°
70	98°
60	97° 36°
50	96° 35.5°

Respirations																									
Blood Pressure																									
Weight																									

	7-3	3-11	11-7	Total	7-3	3-11	11-7	Total	7-3	3-11	11-7	Total	7-3	3-11	11-7	Total	7-3	3-11	11-7	Total
Intake Oral																				
Parenteral																				
Total																				
Output Urine																				
Drainage																				
Emesis																				
Total																				
Stools																				

GRAPHIC CHART

PHYSICIANS' PROGRESS RECORD	

DATE	Note progress of case, complications, consultations, change in diagnosis, condition on discharge, instructions to patient.

NURSES' NOTES AND ACTIVITY FLOW SHEET

DATE _____

INTAKE

IMED									
Solutions/ Amounts						BLOOD PRODUCTS	PO	TUBE FEEDING	FLUIDS PER TUBE
Time	1/	2/	3/	4/	5/				
2400									

2300-0700		

8° Total — IV:
Credit
0800

0700-1500		

8° Total — IV:
Credit
1600

1500-2300		

8° Total — IV:
Credit
24° Total — IV:

24° TOTAL	

BLOOD PRODUCTS

	UNIT #	TIME
1		
2		
3		
4		
5		
6		
7		
8		
9		
10		

SIGNATURES

2300-0700	

0700-1500	

1500-2300	

OUTPUT

Time	Urine	Cath	N.G.	Emesis	C.T.			
2400								

2300-0700	

8° Total
0800

0700-1500	

8° Total
1600

1500-2300	

8° Total
24° Total

24° TOTAL	

CODES (EVALUATION / INTERVENTION)

1. NEW ORDER
2. DC'd, CATH INTACT
3. DRESSING CHANGED
4. TUBING CHANGED
5. ROUTINE SITE ROTATION
6. REDNESS AT SITE
7. SWELLING AT SITE
8. C/O PAIN
9. NO PROBLEM NOTED
10. OTHER (SEE NURSE'S NOTES)

IV MAINTENANCE RECORD

TIME	CODE	CATH SIZE	SITE	# STICKS	E/I	INITIALS

PATIENT RECORD-1

PATIENT NAME _____ DATE _____

	TIME															CODES

CARDIOVASCULAR

HEART Intensity		
RHYTHM		
SKIN		
COLOR		
NAIL BEDS		
CAPILLARY REFILL		
EDEMA		
RADIALS		
PEDALS		
TELEMETRY #		
PACEMAKER Rate		
Type/Mode		

GI

ABDOMEN	
BOWEL SOUNDS	
CIRCUMFERENCE	

NEURO

COMA
EYES	
VERBAL	
MOTOR	

PUPILS
RT	SIZE	
	REAC	
LT	SIZE	
	REAC	

RT	ARMS	
	LEGS	
LT	ARMS	
	LEGS	

FONTANEL	

RESPIRATORY

Respirations (Quality)	
Breath RU	
Sounds RL	
LU	
LL	
O₂ MODE	
Administration LF/FIO₂	

SIGNATURES	

CODES

HEART INTENSITY
WNL- Within Normal
↓ — Muffled-Distant

RHYTHM
R - Regular
IR- Irregular

SKIN
W—Warm
C —Cold
H —Hot
DIA —Diaphoretic
MST—Moist
DR —Dry

COLOR and/or NAILBEDS
FL —Flushed
G —Good, Pink
P —Pale
DSK—Dusky
CY —Cyanotic
J —Jaundiced
ASH—Ashen
T —Tan

CAPILLARY REFILL
< 3 seconds—Normal
> 3 seconds—Sluggish
0—Absent

EDEMA
P —Pitting
NP—Non-pitting

PULSES
R / L
0 —Absent
1 + —Intermittent
2+ —Weak
3 + —Normal
4 + —Strong

TELEMETRY
NSR —Normal Sinus Rhythm
SB —Sinus Bradycardia
SVT —Supraventricular Tachycardia
PVC's —Premature Ventricular Contractions
AF —Atrial Fibrillation
VT —Ventricular Tachycardia
AIVR —Accelerated Idioventricular Rate
PAC's —Premature Atrial Contractions

PACEMAKER
Type:
PM—Permanent
TV —Transvenous
PW—Pacing Wires
Mode:
A—Asynchronous
D—Demand

ABDOMEN
FT —Flat
DIS —Distended
LG —Large
TEN—Tender
ST —Soft, Pliable
FM —Firm
RIG —Rigid

BOWEL SOUNDS
+ —Present
+o —Hypoactive
++ —Hyperactive
o —Absent

COMA SCALE
Eyes Open
4. Spontaneously
3. To speech
2. To pain
1. No response
Verbal Response
5. Oriented
4. Confused
3. Inappropriate
2. Incomprehensive
1. No response
C Crying
Motor Response
6. Obey commands
5. Localizes pain
4. Flexion-withdrawal
3. Flexion-abnormal (decorticate rigidity)
2. Extension to pain (decerebrate rigidity)
1. No response

PEDS COMA SCALE

Verbal Response		
>2 yrs	<2 yrs	
Oriented	Sociable	5
Confused	Consolable cry	4
Inappropriate	Persistent cry	3
Incomprehensible	Agitated	2
None	None	1

Best Motor Response		
Spontaneous	Appropriate for age	6
Localizes to pain		5
Withdraws to pain		4
Flexion to pain (decorticate)		3
Extension to pain (decerebrate)		2
No response		1

PUPIL REACTION
+ —Reacts
− —No reaction
c —Eye closed

PUPIL SCALE (mm)
● ●
1 2
● ● ●
3 4 5
● ● ●
6 7 8

ARMS & LEGS
6. Normal power
5. Mild weakness
4. Severe weakness
3. Spastic flexion
2. Extension
1. No response

RESPIRATIONS
R —Regular
I —Irregular
S —Shallow
L —Labored
RT —Retractions
STR—Stridor

FONTANEL
B —Bulging
F —Flat
SU—Sunken
P —Pulsing
T —Tense
SO—Soft

BREATH SOUNDS
CL—Clear
CR—Crackles
CS—Coarse
RA—Rales
RH—Rhonchi
W —Wheeze
I —Inspiratory
E —Expiratory
D —Decreased
0 —Absent

O₂ MODE
M —Mask
NP —Nasal Prongs
ET —Endotracheal
T —Trach
TN—Tent
H —Hood

PATIENT RECORD - 2

DATE _____

PATIENT CARE	2400						0800						1600						CODES
ISOLATION																			**ISOLATION** AFB—Respiratory BF —Blood & Body Fluids
TURN																			**TURN** R—Right L—Left B—Back
BATH																			**BATH** C —Complete P —Partial PA—Partial/Assist S —Shower SA—Shower/Assist SB—Self Bath T —Tub Bath TA—Tub Assist
ORAL/TRACH CARE																			
PERI/FOLEY CARE																			
ACTIVITY																			**ACTIVITY** BRPA: B —Bedrest A—AROM P—PROM H —Held PR —Playroom BRP —Bathroom Privileges BRPA —with assist BSC —Bedside Commode
BACK CARE																			
LINEN CHANGE																			
↑ SIDERAILS																			BSCA—with assist C —Chair (Self) CA —with assist DA —Dangle/Assist W —Walking WA —Walking/assist S —Sleeping
DIET/APPETITE (% or cc's)																			
EQUIPMENT																			**RESTRAINTS** WRIST: left/right ANKLE: left/right BW —Both Wrists BA —Both Ankles P —Posey CC —Cadillac Chair CCA —with assist 2-3-4
GI TUBE: Placement Checked																			
GI TUBE: Tube type/Suction																			
GI TUBE: Hematest, Color, Char.																			**DIET** FT—Fed Totally FP—Fed Partially TF—Tube Fed
STOOL: Method of Output																			
STOOL: Amt. Description																			**EQUIPMENT** IM —IMED OX—Oximeter KP —Kangaroo Pump AM—Apnea Monitor HO—Hypothermia Blanket HP —Hyperthermia Blanket A —Airshields Warmer IS —Isolette K —K-Pad
STOOL: Hematest																			
URINE: Catheter																			
URINE: Method of Output																			
URINE: Specific Gravity Color, Char.																			
RESP: Rx Chest Pt.																			**STOOL/METHOD** T—Toilet D—Dilly I —Incontinent
RESP: Suctioned																			
RESP: Secretions (color, type, amt.) ET Oral																			**URINE/METHOD** Catheter Size/Date of Insertion D —Diaper BP—Bedpan I —Incontinent
TESTS/PROC: Specimen Sent																			
TESTS/PROC: Procedures																			**PERI/FOLEY CARE** P—Peri F—Foley
TESTS/PROC: Tests/X-rays																			
DRAINS: Site Location																			**DRAINAGE** CL—Clear BL—Bloody S —Serous SS—Serosanguinous T —Tan
DRAINS: Dressing Change																			
WOUND: Site: location/condition																			
WOUND: Dressing Change																			
FLAPS/GRAFTS																			
SIGNATURES																			

PATIENT RECORD - 3

PATIENT NAME _____   DATE _____

NOTIFICATION	TIME	NURSING CONCERNS	RESPONSE TIME/ACTION TAKEN	INIT.

DISCHARGE/TEACHING INSTRUCTIONS

PATIENT BEHAVIORS/OBSERVATIONS/EVALUATION/INTERVENTIONS (NURSES' NOTES)

PATIENT RECORD - 4

HISTORY AND PHYSICAL EXAMINATION

Final Diagnosis: To be recorded when determined_____

_____

Age____Sex_____ Race____ S.M.W. yrs. ____ Adm.____ Dis.____

Family History	Age	Health, if living, or cause of death Note especially Hereditary or Infectious diseases
Father		
Mother		
Brothers		
Sisters		

Chief Complaint: Date and mode of onset, probable cause, course

Past History: Diseases from childhood to date, habits, menstrual history, social data

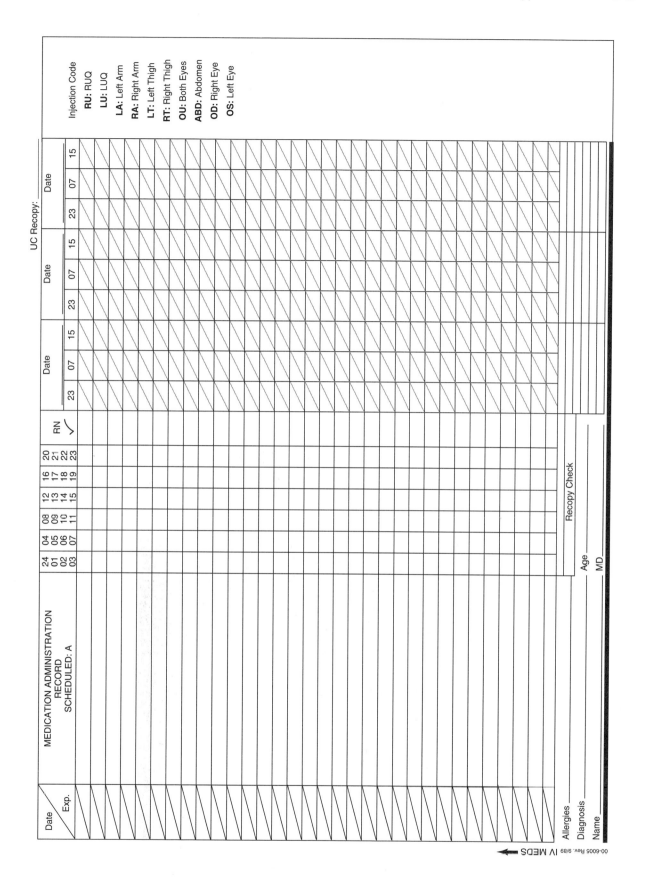

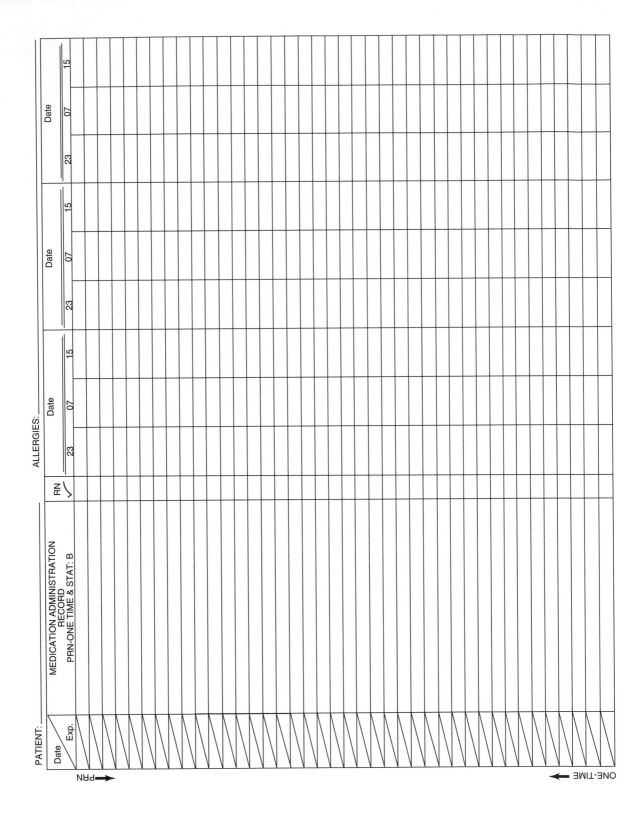

PHYSICIANS' DISCHARGE SUMMARY

Patient Name: _____

MR#: _____

Date of Admission: _____

Date of Discharge: _____

Principle Diagnosis: _____

_____

_____

_____

Secondary Diagnosis: _____

_____

_____

_____

Operations or Procedures:

_____

_____

_____

Brief History and Essential Physical Findings:

_____

_____

_____

_____

_____

Significant Laboratory, X-ray and Consultation Findings:

_____

_____

_____

Course in Hospital with Complications, if any:

_____

_____

_____

Disposition including follow-up treatment, medication by name and dosage, discharge instructions:

_____

_____

_____

_____

_____

_____

Physician's Signature: _____

NURSES' DISCHARGE PLANNING INSTRUCTIONS

DATES OF HOSPITALIZATION   FROM_____ TO_____ DISCHARGE DATE_____ TIME _____

HOSPITAL
DIAGNOSIS: **1.**_____   **2.**_____

3._____   **4.**_____

DIET
INSTRUCTIONS:_____

TREATMENTS:_____

ACTIVITIES:_____

SUPPLIES:_____

MEDICATIONS	STRENGTH	INSTRUCTIONS	PRESCRIPTION GIVEN	
			YES	NO
1.				
2.				
3.				
4.				
5.				
6.				
7.				
8.				

CALL DR._____ OFFICE FOR APPOINTMENT IN/ON_____ _____M.D.

I UNDERSTAND THE ABOVE INSTRUCTIONS   YES ☐   NO ☐   ALL PERSONAL BELONGINGS TAKEN HOME YES ☐   NO ☐

IF NO EXPLAIN_____

DATE_____ TIME_____ PATIENT/RESPONSIBLE PARTY SIGNATURE _____

INDEPENDENT IN ADL YES ☐   NO ☐   ALERT ☐   ORIENTED TO TIME AND PLACE ☐   DISORIENTED ☐
CONFUSED: AT INTERVALS ☐   AT NIGHT ONLY ☐   SEMI-COMATOSE ☐   COMATOSE ☐

DESCRIPTION OF SKIN _____

DESCRIPTION OF INCISION _____
BRIEFLY DESCRIBE ANY PROBLEM IN THE FOLLOWING AREAS:

VISION_____ HEARING _____ SPEECH_____

AMBULATION _____ DEFORMITY_____ PROSTHESIS/EQUIPMENT_____

OTHER _____

MODE OF
DISCHARGE _____ ACCOMPANIED BY_____ DISCHARGE DESTINATION _____

HOME CARE REFERRAL: NO_____YES_____AGENCY_____

DATE _____ RN _____

MR 685-755 (T) REV. 5-80

DISCHARGE INSTRUCTIONS

CHART COPY

Kardex Form

Activity	Date Ord	Treatments	Date Ord	Laboratory	Date Ord	Allergies	
						Diagnostic Imaging	Date to
Diet							be Done
Vital signs							
Weight							
IV		Respiratory Care		Pre OP Orders		Diagnostic Studies	
				Daily Lab			
I & O							
Retention Cath (Foley)		Physical Medicine					
☐ Health Records _____							
Adm. Date		Consultations:		Surgery: Date:			
Name	Doctor		Age	Diagnosis		Date of admission	

Doctor Ordering _____   ☐ Stat
Today's Date _____   ☐ Routine
Requested by _____

Central Service Department

☐ Adult disposable diapers
☐ Alternating pressure pad
☐ Colostomy kit
☐ Colostomy irrigation bag
☐ Egg-crate mattress
☐ Elastic abdominal binder size _____
☐ Footboard
☐ Feeding pump with bag and tubing
☐ Feeding bag and tubing
☐ Footboard
☐ Foot cradle
☐ Hypothermia machine
☐ Isolation pack
☐ IV infusion pump with tubing
☐ K-pad with motor
☐ Nasal gastric tube type _____ size _____
☐ Pleur-evac
☐ Pneumatic Hose
☐ Restraints   type _____

☐ Sitz bath, disposable
☐ Stomal bags type _____ size _____
☐ Suction canister and tubing
☐ Suction catheter type _____ size _____
☐ Ted hose
   ☐ Thigh high   size _____
   ☐ Knee high   size _____
☐ Vaginal irrigation kit

Sterile Trays:

☐ Bone marrow
☐ Central line
☐ Lumbar Puncture (Spinal Tap)
☐ Paracentesis
☐ Thoracentesis
☐ Tracheostomy

☐ Write in item _____
_____

Doctor Ordering _____ ☐ Routine
Today's Date _____ ☐ Stat
Requested by _____

| **Dietary Department** |

☐ Bland
☐ _____Calorie ADA
☐ Calorie count
_____Calorie
☐ Cardiac
☐ Clear liquid
☐ Dietician consult
☐ Early tray
☐ Finger food
☐ Force fluids
☐ Full liquid
☐ Guest tray
☐ Gluten free

☐ Hold tray_____
☐ Kosher
☐ Low cholesterol
☐ Low sodium
☐ Mechanical soft
☐ Modified fat_____
☐ NPO
☐ Pediatric
☐ Protein modified_____g
☐ Prudent cardiac
☐ Pureed
☐ Regular
☐ Release from hold

☐ Renal
☐ Restrict fluids to_____
☐ Snacks/supplements
☐ _____Sodium
☐ Soft
☐ Vegetarian

☐ Other_____

Food allergies_____
Preferences_____
Comments_____

_____
_____
_____

Doctor Ordering _____

Today's Date _____

Collection Date _____ Time _____

Collected by _____

Requested by _____

☐ Stat

☐ Routine

Hematology	**Serology**	**Urinalysis/Urine Chemistry**
☐ Bleeding Time, Ivy	☐ ANA	☐ Routine Ua
☐ CBC c̄ Diff	☐ ASO Titer	☐ Amylase (2hr)
☐ CBC c̄ Manual Diff	☐ CEA	☐ Bilirubin
☐ Factor VIII	☐ CMV	☐ Calcium
☐ Fibrinogen	☐ IgG	☐ Chloride
☐ HCT	☐ IgM	☐ Creatinine Clearance
☐ HGB	☐ Cocci Screen	☐ Glucose Tolerance
☐ H & H	☐ EBV Panel	☐ Nitrogen
☐ Eosinophil Ct Absolute	☐ Enterovirus Ab Panel 1	☐ Occult Blood
☐ Eosinophil Smear	☐ Enterovirus Ab Panel 2	☐ Osmolality
☐ ESR	☐ HbsAb	☐ Phosphorus
☐ LE Cell Prep	☐ HbsAg	☐ Potassium
☐ Platelet Ct	☐ HIV	☐ Pregnancy
☐ PT	☐ Monospot	☐ Protein
☐ PTT (APTT)	☐ PSA Screen	☐ Sodium
☐ RBC	☐ Ra Factor	☐ Sp Gravity
☐ RBC Indices	☐ RPR	☐ Uric Acid
☐ Reticulocyte Ct	☐ RSV	
☐ Sickle Cell Prep	☐ Rubella Screen	
☐ WBC	☐ Strptozyme	
	☐ VDRL	

Write in Orders: _____

_____

Revised 3/12/03

Doctor Ordering _____ ☐ Stat
Today's Date _____ ☐ T/Stat
Collection Date _____ Time _____ ☐ Routine
Collected by _____
Requested by _____

Chemistry

☐ Acetone
☐ Acid phos.
☐ ACE level
☐ ACTH
☐ A/G ratio
☐ Albumin
☐ Aldolase
☐ Alk Phos.
☐ Amylase
☐ ALT (SGPT)
☐ Amino acid screen
☐ Bilirubin, total
   ☐ Direct
   ☐ Indirect
☐ BMP
☐ BNP
☐ BUN
☐ Calcium
☐ Cardiac Enzymes
   ☐ CK (CPK)
   ☐ LDH
   ☐ AST (SGOT)
☐ Citrate
☐ CKMB
☐ CKMB Panel
☐ Cholesterol
☐ CMP
☐ C-reactive Protein
☐ Creatinine

☐ Cortisol
☐ Electrolytes
   ☐ Sodium
   ☐ Potassium
   ☐ Chloride
   ☐ Carbon Dioxide
☐ Folic Acid
☐ Folate
☐ FSH
☐ Glucose
☐ Glucose, _____ Hr PP
☐ Glucose Tolerance _____ Hr
☐ Iron
☐ Lactic Acid
☐ LDH Isoenzymes
☐ LH
☐ Lipase
☐ Magnesium
☐ Osmolality
☐ Phosphorus
☐ Protein
☐ Protein Electrophoresis
☐ TBG
☐ Triglycerides
☐ Troponin
☐ TSH
☐ T_3
☐ T_4
☐ Uric Acid
☐ VMA

Toxicology

☐ Acetaminophen
   ☐ Peak
   ☐ Trough
☐ Aminophylline
   ☐ Peak
   ☐ Trough
☐ Digitoxin
   ☐ Peak
   ☐ Trough
☐ Digoxin
   ☐ Peak
   ☐ Trough
☐ Drug Screen
☐ Gentamycin
   ☐ Peak
   ☐ Trough
☐ Kanamycin
   ☐ Peak
   ☐ Trough
☐ Lidocaine
   ☐ Peak
   ☐ Trough
☐ Phenobarbital
   ☐ Peak
   ☐ Trough
☐ Vancomycin
   ☐ Peak
   ☐ Trough

Write in Orders: _____

Revised 2/4/03

Doctor Ordering _____ ☐ Stat
Today's Date _____ ☐ Routine
Collection Date _____ Time _____
Collected by _____
Requested by _____

Microbiology

Specimen Source	Test Requested
☐ Abscess	☐ AFB Culture
_____	☐ AFB Stain
☐ Blood	☐ C & S
☐ Body Cavity	☐ C & S
_____	Anaerobic
☐ CSF	☐ Fungal Culture
☐ Ear Drainage	☐ GC Screen
☐ Right	☐ Strep Screen
☐ Left	☐ Viral Culture
☐ Eye Drainage	☐ Other
☐ Right	_____
☐ Left	
☐ Nasal Smear	
☐ Sputum	
☐ Stool	☐ Stool
☐ Throat	☐ Fat
☐ Tissue	☐ Fiber
_____	☐ Occult Blood
☐ Urine	☐ Ova & Parasites
☐ Voided	☐ #1 of 3
☐ Clean Catch	☐ #2 of 3
☐ St Cath	☐ #3 of 3
☐ Foley Cath	
☐ Wound Drainage _____	
☐ Other _____	

Fluids

Specimen Source	Test Requested
☐ Abdominal	☐ Cell Count
☐ Amniotic	c̄ Diff
☐ CSF	☐ Glucose
☐ Pericardial	☐ LDH
☐ Peritoneal	☐ Occult Blood
☐ Pleural	☐ Protein
☐ Synovial	☐ Sp Gravity
☐ Other	☐ VDRL (CSF)
# of Tubes _____	☐ Other
	_____

Cytology

Specimen Source	Test Requested
☐ Amniotic	☐ Pap
☐ Breast Bx	☐ Fungal
☐ Bronchial Asp	☐ Buccal
☐ Cervical Smear	☐ Maturation
☐ Cervical Bx	Index
☐ Colon Bx	☐ Other_____
☐ CSF	
☐ Gastric Fluid	
☐ Lung Asp	
☐ Pleural	
☐ Pericardial	
☐ Peritoneal	
☐ Sputum	
☐ Vaginal	
☐ Other _____	

Revised 3/11/03

Doctor Ordering _____ ☐ Stat
Today's Date _____ ☐ Routine
Collection Date _____ Time _____
Collected by _____
Requested by _____

Blood Bank

☐ Routine   ☐ ASAP   ☐ Stat   ☐ For Hold
_____

Date of Surgery_____ Date of Transfusion _____

                                                                       # of Units

Autologous Blood?   yes ___ no ___   ☐ Whole Blood   _____
Donor Specific?   yes ___ no ___   ☐ Packed Cells   _____
☐ Type and X-match   ☐ Washed Cells   _____
☐ Type and Screen   ☐ Frozen Cells   _____
                                               ☐ Fresh Frozen Plasma _____
☐ Coombs Test   ☐ Platelet Concentrate _____
☐ Other_____   ☐ Cryoprecipitate   _____
                                               ☐ Other_____

Comments _____
_____
_____

Revised 3/11/03

CONSENT TO OPERATION, ADMINISTRATION OF ANESTHETICS, AND THE RENDERING OF OTHER MEDICAL SERVICES

1. I authorize and direct _____ M.D., my surgeon and/or associates or assistants of his choice, to perform the following operation upon me

_____

and/or to do any other therapeutic procedure that (his) (their) judgment may dictate to be advisable for the patient's well-being. The nature of the operation has been explained to me and no warranty or guarantee has been made as to the result or cure.

2. I hereby authorize and direct the above-named surgeon and/or his associates or assistants to provide such additional services for me as he or they may deem reasonable and necessary, including, but not limited to, the administration and maintenance of the anesthesia, and the performance of services involving pathology and radiology, and I hereby consent thereto.

3. I understand that the above-named surgeon and his associates or assistants will be occupied solely with performing such operation, and the persons in attendance at such operation for the purpose of administering anesthesia, and the person or persons performing services involving pathology and radiology, are not the agents, servants or employees of the above named hospital nor of any surgeon, but are independent contractors.

4. Permission for observation of operation for visiting M.D.'s, nurses, medical students, interns and residents is hereby granted at the discretion of the physician in charge, subject to current rules and regulations of the hospital.

5. I hereby authorize the hospital pathologist to use his discretion in the disposal of any severed tissue

or member, except _____

_____   _____   _____
(PATIENT)   (WITNESS)   (TIME & DATE)

(If patient is a minor or unable to sign, complete the following:)

Patient is a minor _____, or is unable to sign, because _____

_____

_____   _____   _____
(FATHER/MOTHER)   (WITNESS)   (TIME & DATE)

_____   _____   _____
(OTHER PERSON & RELATIONSHIP)   (WITNESS)   (TIME & DATE)

CONSENT TO OPERATION

CONSENT FOR TRANSFUSION(S)

1. I authorize the administration of such transfusions of whole blood or blood products to the above patients as may be deemed advisable in the judgment of the patient's attending physician, his associates or assistants.

2. It has been fully explained to me and I understand that blood transfusions are not always successful in producing a desirable result. It has also been explained to me and I understand that despite the exercise of due care, the transfusion of blood or blood products is always attended with a possibility of some ill effects, such as: the transmission of hepatitis; accidental immunization; allergic reactions; or in rare instances Acquired Immune Deficiency Syndrome (AIDS).

3. It has also been explained to me and I understand that emergencies do, on occasion, arise when it may be necessary for the patient's well being to use existing stocks of blood which may not include the most compatible blood types.

4. **I UNDERSTAND AND AGREE THAT NO GUARANTEE OR WARRANTY (INCLUDING THE IMPLIED WARRANTIES OF MERCHANTABILITY AND FITNESS) APPLIES TO THE BLOOD OR BLOOD PRODUCTS WHICH MAY BE SUPPLIED TO THIS PATIENT.**

5. I accept on behalf of this patient all of the risks referred to above.

_____   _____
Patient   **Witness**

_____   _____
Person Authorized to Sign for Patient   **Date**

_____
Relationship

_____
Reason for signature by person authorized to sign for patient in lieu of, or in addition to, signature by patient.

Consent For Transfusion Of Blood Or Blood Products

1. I HAVE BEEN INFORMED that I need or may need during treatment, a transfusion of blood and/or one of its products in the interest of my health and proper medical care.

2. I HAVE BEEN INFORMED of the risks and benefits of receiving transfusion(s). These risks exist despite the fact that the blood has been carefully tested.

3. The alternatives to transfusion, including the risks and consequences of not receiving this therapy, have been explained to me.

4. I have read, or had read to me, the Blood Transfusion Information regarding blood transfusions and have had the opportunity to ask questions.

5. I hereby consent to the transfusion(s).

| _____ | _____ | _____ |
| Patient's Signature | Date | Time |

Signature of parent, legally appointed guardian or responsible person
(for patients who cannot sign)

| _____ | _____ | _____ |
| Witness | Date | Time |

Refusal To Permit Blood Transfusion

1. I request that no blood derivatives be administered to ⸺⸺⸺⸺⸺⸺⸺
   during this hospitalization.　　　　　　　　　　(patient name)

2. I hereby release the hospital, its personnel and the attending physician from any responsibility whatever for unfavorable reactions or any untoward results due to my refusal to permit the use of blood or its derivatives.

3. I fully understand the possible consequences of such refusal on my part.

_____　　_____　　_____
Patient's Signature　　　　　　　　　Date　　　　　　　　　　　Time

Signature of parent, legally appointed guardian or responsible person
(for patients who cannot sign)

_____　　_____　　_____
Witness　　　　　　　　　　　　Date　　　　　　　　　　　Time

_____　　_____　　_____
Witness　　　　　　　　　　　　Date　　　　　　　　　　　Time

Doctor Ordering _____

Date to be done _____ ☐ Stat ☐ Routine ☐ ASAP

Today's Date _____ Requested by _____

Diagnostic Imaging - X-Ray Procedures

Clinical Indication _____

Transportation ☐ portable ☐ stretcher ☐ wheelchair ☐ ambulatory

O$_2$ ☐ yes ☐ no	Diabetic ☐ yes ☐ no	Hearing deficit ☐ yes ☐ no
IV ☐ yes ☐ no	Seizure disorder ☐ yes ☐ no	Sight deficit ☐ yes ☐ no
Isolation ☐ yes ☐ no	Non-English speaking ☐ yes ☐ no	

Comments: _____

☐ Abdomen _____

☐ Bone x-ray order: _____

☐ Chest order: _____

☐ KUB order: _____

☐ Mammogram _____

☐ Sinus series order: _____

☐ SNAT series _____

☐ Spine order: _____

☐ BE _____

☐ GB _____

☐ IVU _____

☐ SBFT _____

☐ UGI _____

☐ Write in order _____

_____

_____

_____

Doctor Ordering _____

Date to be done _____ ☐ Stat ☐ Routine ☐ ASAP

Today's Date _____ Requested by _____

| **Diagnostic Imaging—Special Procedures** |

Clinical Indication _____

Transportation ☐ portable ☐ stretcher ☐ wheelchair ☐ ambulatory

O$_2$ ☐ yes ☐ no   Diabetic ☐ yes ☐ no   Hearing deficit ☐ yes ☐ no

IV ☐ yes ☐ no   Seizure disorder ☐ yes ☐ no   Sight deficit ☐ yes ☐ no

Isolation ☐ yes ☐ no   Non-English speaking ☐ yes ☐ no

Comments: _____

☐ Abdominal arteriogram _____

☐ Arthrogram _____

☐ Cerebral angiogram _____

☐ Cervical myelogram _____

☐ Hysterosalpingogram _____

☐ Lymphangiogram _____

☐ Spinal myelogram _____

☐ Venogram _____

☐ Voiding cystourethrogram _____

☐ Write in order _____

_____

_____

_____

Doctor Ordering _____

Date to be done _____ ☐ Stat ☐ Routine ☐ ASAP

Today's Date _____ Requested by_____

Diagnostic Imaging—Computed Tomography

Clinical Indication _____

☐ with contrast   ☐ without contrast

Transportation ☐ portable ☐ stretcher ☐ wheelchair ☐ ambulatory

O_2 ☐ yes ☐ no	Diabetic ☐ yes ☐ no	Hearing deficit ☐ yes ☐ no
IV ☐ yes ☐ no	Seizure disorder ☐ yes ☐ no	Sight deficit ☐ yes ☐ no
Isolation ☐ yes ☐ no	Non-English speaking ☐ yes ☐ no	

Comments:_____

☐ CT scan of head _____

☐ CT scan of brain _____

☐ CT scan of abdomen _____

☐ CT scan of pelvis _____

☐ CT scan of spine _____

☐ CT of neck _____

☐ CT guided liver biopsy _____

☐ Write in order _____

_____

_____

_____

Doctor Ordering _____

Date to be done _____ □ Stat □ Routine □ ASAP

Today's Date _____ Requested by _____

Diagnostic Imaging—Ultrasonography

Clinical Indication _____

Transportation □ portable □ stretcher □ wheelchair □ ambulatory

O_2 □ yes □ no	Diabetic □ yes □ no	Hearing deficit □ yes □ no
IV □ yes □ no	Seizure disorder □ yes □ no	Sight deficit □ yes □ no
Isolation □ yes □ no	Non-English speaking □ yes □ no	

Comments: _____

□ US of abd _____

□ US of pelvis _____

□ US of GB _____

□ Write in order _____

_____

_____

_____

Doctor Ordering _____

Date to be done _____ ☐ Stat ☐ Routine ☐ ASAP

Today's Date _____ Requested by _____

Diagnostic Imaging—Magnetic Resonance Imaging

Clinical Indication _____

Transportation ☐ portable ☐ stretcher ☐ wheelchair ☐ ambulatory

O_2 ☐ yes ☐ no   Diabetic ☐ yes ☐ no   Hearing deficit ☐ yes ☐ no

IV ☐ yes ☐ no   Seizure disorder ☐ yes ☐ no   Sight deficit ☐ yes ☐ no

Isolation ☐ yes ☐ no   Non-English speaking ☐ yes ☐ no

Comments: _____

☐ MRI of brain _____

☐ MRI of spine _____

☐ MRI shoulder _____

☐ MRI knee _____

☐ Write in order _____

_____

_____

_____

Doctor Ordering_____

Date to be done_____ ☐ Stat ☐ Routine ☐ ASAP

Today's Date_____ Requested by_____

Diagnostic Imaging—Nuclear Medicine

Clinical Indication_____

Transportation ☐ portable ☐ stretcher ☐ wheelchair ☐ ambulatory

O₂ ☐ yes ☐ no   Diabetic ☐ yes ☐ no   Hearing deficit ☐ yes ☐ no

IV ☐ yes ☐ no   Seizure disorder ☐ yes ☐ no   Sight deficit ☐ yes ☐ no

Isolation ☐ yes ☐ no   Non-English speaking ☐ yes ☐ no

Comments: _____

☐ Bone scan (total)_____

☐ Bone scan (regional)_____

☐ Liver and spleen_____

☐ Gallium scan_____

☐ Thyroid uptake and scan_____

☐ DISIDA_____

☐ PET_____

☐ MUGA_____

☐ Thallium stress scan_____

☐ Adenosine/thallium scan_____

☐ Sestamibi stress_____

☐ Write in order_____

_____

_____

_____

Doctor Ordering_____

Date to be done_____ ☐ Stat ☐ Routine ☐ ASAP

Today's Date_____ Requested by_____

| **Cardiovascular Department** |

Clinical Indication _____

Cardiac Medications _____

Pacemaker? ☐ yes ☐ no   Type _____   Ht_____ Wt_____

Comments: _____

LOC? ☐ yes ☐ no

Noninvasive Studies

☐ Cardiac monitor

☐ Carotid Doppler flow analysis

☐ Carotid phonoangiography

☐ Doppler flow studies _____

☐ Echocardiogram 2D M-Mode

☐ EKG

☐ EKG c̄ Rhythm Strip

☐ Holter monitor_____hours

☐ Impedance plethysmography
   studies_____

☐ Transesophageal electrocardiogram

☐ Treadmill stress test

Invasive Studies

☐ Cardiac catheterization

☐ Write in order_____

☐ Electrophysiological Studies

Transportation ☐ portable ☐ stretcher ☐ wheelchair ☐ ambulatory

O₂ ☐ yes ☐ no   Diabetic ☐ yes ☐ no   Hearing deficit ☐ yes ☐ no

IV ☐ yes ☐ no   Seizure disorder ☐ yes ☐ no   Sight deficit ☐ yes ☐ no

Isolation ☐ yes ☐ no   Non-English speaking ☐ yes ☐ no

Doctor Ordering_____

Date to be done_____ ☐ Stat ☐ Routine ☐ ASAP

Today's Date _____ Requested by_____

Neurodiagnostics Department

Clinical Indication _____

Transportation ☐ portable ☐ stretcher ☐ wheelchair ☐ ambulatory

O₂ ☐ yes ☐ no	Diabetic ☐ yes ☐ no	Hearing deficit ☐ yes ☐ no
IV ☐ yes ☐ no	Seizure disorder ☐ yes ☐ no	Sight deficit ☐ yes ☐ no
Isolation ☐ yes ☐ no	Non-English speaking ☐ yes ☐ no	

Comments: _____

☐ Auditory Evoked Response
☐ Echoencephalography
☐ Electroencephalography
☐ Electromyography
☐ Electronystagmography
☐ Nerve Conduction Studies
☐ Somatosensory Evoked Potential
☐ Visual Evoked Potential

Write in order _____

_____

_____

_____

Doctor Ordering_____

Date to be done_____ Time to be done_____

Today's Date _____ Requested by_____

Endoscopy Department

Clinical Indication_____

Transportation ☐ portable ☐ stretcher ☐ wheelchair ☐ ambulatory

O$_2$ ☐ yes ☐ no   Diabetic ☐ yes ☐ no   Hearing deficit ☐ yes ☐ no

IV ☐ yes ☐ no   Seizure disorder ☐ yes ☐ no   Sight deficit ☐ yes ☐ no

Isolation ☐ yes ☐ no   Non-English speaking ☐ yes ☐ no

Pre-op Medication ☐ yes ☐ no

Time given _____

Comments: _____

☐ Arthroscopy   ☐ Esophagoscopy

☐ Bronchoscopy   ☐ Hysteroscopy

☐ Colonoscopy   ☐ Laparoscopy

☐ Colposcopy   ☐ Pelvioscopy

☐ Cystoscopy   ☐ Peritoneoscopy

☐ Endoscopic retrograde   ☐ Proctoscopy
   cholangiopancreatography (ERCP)   ☐ Sigmoidoscopy

☐ Esophagogastroduodenoscopy (EGD)

☐ Write in order _____

_____

_____

_____

Doctor Ordering_____

Date to be done _____ ☐ Stat ☐ Routine ☐ ASAP

Today's Date _____ Requested by _____

Respiratory Care Department—Diagnostics

Clinical Indication _____

Anticoagulant Medication? ☐ yes Name of medication _____
                          ☐ no

Room air ☐ yes ☐ no   Oxygen ☐ yes ☐ no

Comments: _____

☐ Arterial Blood Gases
☐ Capillary Blood Gases
☐ Pulse oximetry
☐ Spirometry
☐ Write in order_____
  _____
  _____
  _____

Doctor Ordering _____

Date to be done _____ ☐ Stat ☐ Routine ☐ ASAP

Today's Date _____ Requested by _____

Respiratory Care Department Treatments

Clinical Indication _____

Comments: _____

☐ O$_2$ _____ L/M   ☐ NP   ☐ Mask   ☐ Tent   ☐ Other _____

☐ SVN _____

☐ CPT _____

☐ IPPB _____

☐ Incentive spirometry _____

☐ USN _____

☐ HA _____

☐ Bi PAP _____

☐ CPAP _____

Write-in order _____

Ventilator orders

IMV mode _____ TV _____ FIO$_2$ _____ PO$_2$ _____ PS _____ Peep _____

Write-in order _____

Doctor Ordering_____
☐ Stat ☐ Routine ☐ ASAP
Today's Date_____ Requested by_____

Orthopedic Equipment

Diagnosis_____

Comments: _____

☐ Bucks Traction_____
☐ Cervical Traction_____
☐ Traction by Gravity_____
☐ Skin Traction_____
☐ Overhead Frame and Trapeze
☐ Braun Frame
☐ Write in order_____
_____
_____
_____

The Clinical Evaluation Record

The main purpose of the Clinical Evaluation Record is to measure and record the student's performance on the nursing unit. The Clinical Evaluation Record is divided into seven units; the first six are sequenced according to the increasing degree of knowledge and skill the student needs to complete the unit. The objectives and corresponding activities will assist the student in mastering each of the skills required to complete the tasks. A rating scale is provided to measure and record the student's performance level.

The Clinical Evaluation Record tells the student, the instructor, and the preceptor exactly what is expected of the student during his or her clinical experience. Use of this record allows the student to pursue mastery of skills and to arrange an evaluation of skills by the instructor or preceptor. The completed appendix becomes a written record of the student's performance in the clinical setting. The appendix may be used by the instructor to assign grades, or by the student to obtain employment. As with the rest of this book, this appendix corresponds with the textbook, *Health Unit Coordinating*, 5th edition.

To ensure overall competence of student performance, the following course requirements are recommended. To successfully complete the health unit coordinator clinical experience, the student must

1. Perform the tasks listed in this appendix with a rating of C.

2. Have no more than _____ hours of unexcused absences.

3. Behave in an ethical manner and not in any way jeopardize the safety or welfare of patients or coworkers.

4. Demonstrate the ability to form interpersonal relationships with other hospital employees necessary for the delivery of quality patient care.

5. Accept feedback from the instructor and health care facility staff and make behavioral changes requested by the instructor.

6. Demonstrate the ability to function during stressful situations on the nursing unit.

Contents

UNIT 6: TRANSCRIPTION OF DOCTOR'S ORDERS

UNIT 7: HEALTH UNIT COORDINATING PROCEDURES

UNIT 8: ORGANIZATION AND PRIORITIZING SKILLS

The Evaluator's Role

The Clinical Evaluation Record clearly outlines for the student the activities he or she must complete or perform to master the objectives for each unit. The student should notify the instructor or preceptor when ready to be evaluated in performing a task. Performance should be recorded on the rating scale as follows:

C indicates competency, or that the student is able to perform the activity with minimal or no assistance in a manner that would qualify him or her for employment as a health unit coordinator in a health care facility.

N indicates that further practice is needed to demonstrate competency, or that the student was unable to perform the task with minimal or no assistance in a manner that would qualify him or her for employment as a health unit coordinator in a health care facility. Reasons for an *N* rating and remedial activities should be outlined to the student.

A blank space has been left in each unit objective description to specify a date by which the student should complete the unit. To use the Clinical Evaluation Record to its full potential, we suggest that the student cross out procedural steps not used in his or her clinical setting and write in steps that are used but not included here in the spaces provided.

The Student's Role

The Clinical Evaluation Record contains objectives for all the tasks you must perform in order to complete the clinical course. To assist you in completing the objectives, we have included Student Activity Sheets. Some of the activities require you to answer questions in writing. After you have completed these activities, give them to your instructor for evaluation. If they are satisfactory, the instructor will circle *C* on the rating scale. If they are not satisfactory, the instructor will circle *N* on the rating scale. Other activities require your instructor or preceptor to observe your performance. You may practice these activities as often as necessary to achieve competency. When you are ready to have your performance evaluated, ask your instructor or preceptor to observe you while you are performing the activity. If you perform the activity satisfactorily, the instructor will circle *C* on the rating scale. If your performance is less than satisfactory, your instructor will circle *N* on the rating scale. Reasons for an *N* rating and remedial activities will be outlined for you by your instructor.

The units are sequenced according to the increasing degree of skill required to perform the activity; however, you do not need to progress according to the units. Become familiar with the entire appendix. Perform the activities as you are ready and as the opportunity presents itself. The only requirement is that you complete the activities satisfactorily by the end of your clinical experience.

The Clinical Evaluation Record allows you to plan your own clinical activities and to judge your own performance of health unit coordinator tasks. It also becomes a written record of your progress throughout the clinical experience.

The following activities are designed to help you meet the objectives for this unit. You will need to be evaluated by your instructor or preceptor as you perform the activities. Each activity should be completed with a *C* score by the end of the week of the clinical session.

To use the Clinical Evaluation Record to its full potential, we suggest that the student cross out procedural steps not used in his or her clinical setting and write in steps that are used but not included here in the spaces provided.

UNIT 1

Introduction to the Health Care Facility

The following activities are designed to help you meet the objectives for this unit. You will need to be evaluated by your preceptor or instructor as you perform the activity. Each activity should be completed with a *C* (competent) score by the end of the first week of the clinical session.

Objective 1: Locate the following on the nursing unit:	Evaluation		Initials
Kitchen	C	N	_____
Clean utility room	C	N	_____
Dirty utility room	C	N	_____
Medication room	C	N	_____
Report room	C	N	_____

CSD closet	C	N	_____
Linen closet	C	N	_____
Pneumatic tube	C	N	_____
Code cart	C	N	_____
Fire extinguisher	C	N	_____
Telephone code button	C	N	_____
Shredder (if applicable)	C	N	_____
Fax machine	C	N	_____
Label maker (if applicable)	C	N	_____
Admission packet	C	N	_____
Surgery packet	C	N	_____
Supplemental forms	C	N	_____

Objective 2: Write the names of the following health care personnel on the nursing unit

Health unit coordinator _____

Nurse (clinical) manager _____

Team leader (if applicable) _____

Shift manager _____

Staff nurses _____

Certified nursing assistants _____

Other _____

Objective 3: Describe the duties of the health care personnel listed above.

Health unit coordinator _____

Nurse (clinical) manager _____

Team leader (if applicable) _____

Shift manager _____

Staff nurses _____

Certified nursing assistants _____

Other _____

Objective 4: Write the name of the services provided by the nursing unit (e.g., Medical, Pediatrics).

_____   C   N   _____

Objective 5: Locate the following departments in the hospital.

Nursing Administration Office	C N	_____
Staffing Office	C N	_____
Human Resources	C N	_____
Employee Health	C N	_____
Cafeteria	C N	_____
Admitting Department	C N	_____
Health Records Department (Medical Records)	C N	_____
Pharmacy Department	C N	_____
Laboratory Department	C N	_____
Diagnostic Imaging Department	C N	_____
Cardiopulmonary Department (Respiratory/Pulmonary)	C N	_____
Neurodiagnostic Department	C N	_____
Physical and Occupational Therapy Departments	C N	_____
Morgue	C N	_____
Other _____	C N	_____

Objective 6: Demonstrate the use of the pneumatic tube system for conveying devices by sending a tube or conveyor to another area of the hospital.   C   N   _____

Objective 7: Demonstrate the assembly and labeling of a patient's chart.   C   N   _____

Objective 8: Locate the area where patient care forms are stored.   C   N   _____

Objective 9: Identify the standard forms used to prepare a patient's chart at the time of admission to the unit.   C   N   _____

Objective 10: Collect a sample of the following supplemental forms.

Parenteral fluid record form	C	N	_____
Therapy record forms for various departments	C	N	_____
Frequent vital signs record form	C	N	_____
Diabetic, anticoagulant, or other flow sheet	C	N	_____
Surgical consent form	C	N	_____
Consent for blood transfusion	C	N	_____

Objective 11: List other supplemental forms used on the nursing unit.

C	N	_____
C	N	_____

Objective 12: Locate the area on the nursing unit where the central service department supplies are stored.

C	N	_____

List 10 items stored on your unit.

1. _____	C	N	_____
2. _____	C	N	_____
3. _____	C	N	_____
4. _____	C	N	_____
5. _____	C	N	_____
6. _____	C	N	_____
7. _____	C	N	_____
8. _____	C	N	_____
9. _____	C	N	_____
10. _____	C	N	_____

Objective 13: Locate the following resource materials on the nursing unit (may be computerized or hard copy).

PDR/Nursing Drug Handbook	C	N	_____
Medical dictionary	C	N	_____
Policy/procedure manual	C	N	_____

Disaster manual	C	N	_____
Laboratory manual	C	N	_____
Diagnostic imaging manual	C	N	_____
Web site for Human Resources	C	N	_____
Other _____	C	N	_____

Objective 14: Locate the surgery schedule for your nursing unit and identify which patients from your floor are scheduled for surgery.

_____	C	N	_____

Performance Acceptable ☐

Additional Practice and Re-evaluation Needed ☐

Recommendations to Improve Performance: _____

_____

_____

_____

Preceptor's Comments: _____

_____

_____

_____

Instructor's Comments: _____

_____

_____

_____

Student's Comments: _____

_____

_____

_____

UNIT 2
Health Unit Coordinator Communication Skills and Professionalism

The following activities are designed to help you meet the objectives for this unit. You will need to be evaluated by your preceptor or instructor as you perform the activities. Each activity should be completed with a *C* (competent) score by the end of the clinical session.

Objective 1: Demonstrate communication skills.	Evaluation		Initials
Communicate with patients, visitors, and staff in a professional and empathetic manner.	C	N	_____
Communicate admissions/discharges/transfers to nursing staff and admitting department in a timely manner.	C	N	_____
Contact physicians, ancillary services, and other departments as requested.	C	N	_____
Use problem-solving techniques to resolve conflicts.	C	N	_____
Familiarize self with staff and staff assignments.	C	N	_____
Listen to the change-of-shift report and take notes as needed.	C	N	_____
Demonstrate sensitivity to cultural diversity.	C	N	_____
Respond to difficult situations using assertiveness skills.	C	N	_____
Demonstrate coping techniques in stressful situations.	C	N	_____

Objective 2: Demonstrate professional standards.			
Arrive on time prior to the beginning of your shift, prepared to work.	C	N	_____
If unable to attend your clinical session:			
Notify the nursing unit at least 2 hours prior to the start of assigned shift.	C	N	_____
Notify your instructor at least 2 hours prior to the start of assigned shift.	C	N	_____
Take assigned breaks without exceeding time; plan to be on nursing unit at all other times.	C	N	_____
Conform to the dress code outlined by hospital or school program.	C	N	_____
Wear name tag.	C	N	_____
Wear minimum amount of jewelry.	C	N	_____
Display courtesy and professionalism at all times.	C	N	_____
Complete tasks accurately and in a timely manner.	C	N	_____

Utilize free time to enhance job performance by familiarizing
self with unit and department manuals.   C   N   _____

Performance Acceptable ☐

Additional Practice and Re-evaluation Needed ☐

Recommendations to Improve Performance: _____

_____

_____

_____

Preceptor's Comments: _____

_____

_____

_____

Instructor's Comments: _____

_____

_____

_____

Student's Comments: _____

_____

_____

_____

UNIT 3

Communication Devices

The following activities are designed to help you meet the objectives for this unit. You will need to be evaluated by your preceptor or instructor as you perform the activities. Each activity should be completed with a C (competent) score by the end of the clinical session.

Objective 1: Demonstrate effective telephone communication skills when answering incoming calls.

	Evaluation		Initials
Answer the telephone as quickly as possible.	C	N	_____

Excuse yourself, if necessary, from conversations within the nursing
unit prior to answering the telephone.　　　C　　N　　_____

Identify the nursing unit, your name, and your title.　　　C　　N　　_____

Have a pencil and paper at hand to record pertinent information.　　　C　　N　　_____

Speak clearly and distinctly, using a pleasant tone.　　　C　　N　　_____

Ask pertinent questions to establish the caller's identity.　　　C　　N　　_____

Refer all calls regarding a patient's care, status, and so forth to the preceptor or nurse.　　　C　　N　　_____

Communicate the caller's name, the nature of the call, and the
telephone number to the person to whom the call is being referred.　　　C　　N　　_____

Use the "hold button" when required to leave the caller.　　　C　　N　　_____

Objective 2: Demonstrate effective telephone communication skills when placing outgoing calls.

Plan the conversation prior to placing the call by gathering all
of the information pertinent to the call.　　　C　　N　　_____

Identify yourself to the person receiving the call by naming the
hospital, the nursing unit, and your own name and title.　　　C　　N　　_____

Objective 3: Demonstrate effective telephone communication skills when leaving a voice mail message.

Speak slowly and distinctly.　　　C　　N　　_____

If the message includes a name, give the first and last name
and spell the last name.　　　C　　N　　_____

If the message includes numbers, repeat the number at the
beginning and at the end of the message.　　　C　　N　　_____

Objective 4: Demonstrate effective telephone communication skills when paging.

Demonstrate the use of a digital pager by paging your instructor.　　　C　　N　　_____

Page hospital personnel as requested to do so　　　C　　N　　_____

Objective 5: Demonstrate the use of fax machine by faxing pharmacy copies.

　　　C　　N　　_____

Objective 6: Demonstrate appropriate communication skills using the intercom.

Demonstrate use of the intercom to initiate and receive calls speaking in a soft voice.　　　C　　N　　_____

Use discretion when transmitting information via the intercom
to avoid patient embarrassment or alarm.　　　C　　N　　_____

Objective 7: Demonstrate required computer skills.

Sign on to the computer using assigned code.	C	N	_____
Sign off of computer when leaving the nursing unit.	C	N	_____
Demonstrate appropriate use of e-mail.	C	N	_____
Locate doctor's name and telephone number from computerized doctor's roster.	C	N	_____
Locate a patient on another unit by name.	C	N	_____
Locate all pending orders on a patient on your unit.	C	N	_____
Locate lab results on a patient on your unit.	C	N	_____
Order supplies from the supply purchasing department.	C	N	_____
Print a census from your unit.	C	N	_____
Enter newly admitted patient demographic information.	C	N	_____

Performance Acceptable ☐

Additional Practice and Re-evaluation Needed ☐

Recommendations to Improve Performance: _____

_____

_____

_____

Preceptor's Comments: _____

_____

_____

_____

Instructor's Comments: _____

_____

_____

_____

Student's Comments: _____

_____

_____

_____

UNIT 4

Legalities and Confidentiality Dealing with Patient Information

The following activities are designed to help you meet the objectives for this unit. You will need to be evaluated by your preceptor or instructor as you perform the activities. Each activity should be completed with a *C* (competent) score by the end of the clinical session.

Objective 1: Demonstrate knowledge and application of the Health Insurance Portability and Accountability Act (HIPAA) requirements.

	Evaluation		Initials
Discuss patient information only when required to do so for patient care purposes, and in the confines of the nursing unit.	C	N	_____
Allow only authorized health care personnel access to patient charts.	C	N	_____
Copy patient chart forms only when requested to do so in a doctor's order and only after checking the hospital policy on copying patient chart forms.	C	N	_____
Give out information only when instructed to do so by authorized nursing personnel.	C	N	_____

Objective 2: Demonstrate the following legal guidelines when dealing with patient charts and legal documents.

Write accurately and legibly when preparing a surgical consent.	C	N	_____
Do not obliterate or white out information on a legal document.	C	N	_____

Performance Acceptable ☐

Additional Practice and Re-evaluation Needed ☐

Recommendations to Improve Performance: _____

_____

_____

_____

Preceptor's Comments: _____

_____

_____

_____

Instructor's Comments: _____

_____

_____

_____

Student's Comments: _____

_____

_____

_____

UNIT 5

Routine Health Unit Coordinator Tasks

The following activities are designed to help you meet the objectives for this unit. The objectives of this unit are "performance objectives." You will be evaluated by your instructor or preceptor as you perform the activities. Each activity should be completed with a C score by the end of the week of the clinical experience.

	Evaluation		Initials
Objective 1: Given a written set of 20 or more vital signs, graph the temperature, pulse, and respiration (TPR) and blood pressure (BP) on patients' graphic sheets.	C	N	_____
Objective 2: Order daily diagnostic tests for the patients on your unit.	C	N	_____
Objective 3: Given admission, transfer, and discharge data, record these data on the daily census record.	C	N	_____
Objective 4: File diagnostic reports in the patients' charts. Compare the patient's name on the diagnostic report with the patient's name on the back of the chart.	C	N	_____

Performance Acceptable ☐

Additional Practice and Re-evaluation Needed ☐

Recommendations to Improve Performance: _____

_____

_____

_____

Preceptor's Comments: _____

_____

_____

_____

Instructor's Comments: _____

_____

_____

_____

Student's Comments: _____

_____

_____

_____

UNIT 6

Transcription of Physicians' Orders

The following activities are designed to help you meet the objectives for this unit. You will need to be evaluated by your preceptor or instructor as you perform the activities. Each activity should be completed with a *C* (competent) score by the end of the clinical session.

Objective 1: Transcribe activity, positioning, and nursing observation orders.

	Evaluation		Initials
Bathroom privileges (BRP)	C	N	_____
Absolute bedrest (ABR)	C	N	_____
Head of bed elevated thirty degrees (HOB ↑ 30°)	C	N	_____
Intake and output (I & O)	C	N	_____
Vital signs order (VS)	C	N	_____

Pulse oximetry	C	N	_____
Other _____	C	N	_____

Objective 2: Transcribe nursing treatment orders.

Catheterization order	C	N	_____
Enema order	C	N	_____
Blood transfusion order	C	N	_____
Other _____	C	N	_____

Objective 3: Transcribe dietary orders.

Regular diet	C	N	_____
Soft diet	C	N	_____
Clear liquid	C	N	_____
Full liquid	C	N	_____
Total parenteral nutrition (TPN)	C	N	_____
Other _____	C	N	_____

Objective 4: Transcribe medication orders.

Type

Antiinfective	C	N	_____
Narcotic	C	N	_____
Hypnotic	C	N	_____
Antiarrhythmic	C	N	_____
Anticoagulant	C	N	_____
Other _____	C	N	_____

Frequency

Whenever necessary (prn)	C	N	_____
Daily (qd)	C	N	_____
Twice a day (bid)	C	N	_____
Three times a day (tid)	C	N	_____

Four times a day (qid)	C	N	_____
Every 6 hours (q 6 hr)	C	N	_____
Every _____ hours	C	N	_____
Immediately (stat)	C	N	_____
One time only	C	N	_____
Discontinue medication order (DC)	C	N	_____
Change in medication order	C	N	_____
Renewal of medication order	C	N	_____

Objective 5: Transcribe laboratory orders.

Hematology

Complete blood cell count (CBC)	C	N	_____
Prothrombin time (PT)	C	N	_____
Hemoglobin and Hematocrit (H & H)	C	N	_____
Other _____	C	N	_____

Chemistry

Electrolytes (Lytes)	C	N	_____
Comprehensive metabolic panel (CMP)	C	N	_____
Basic metabolic panel (BMP)	C	N	_____
Fasting blood sugar (FBS)	C	N	_____
Two hour post prandial blood sugar (2 hr PP BS)	C	N	_____
Medication Peak & Trough	C	N	_____
Other _____	C	N	_____

Microbiology

Blood cultures	C	N	_____
Stool for ova and parasites (O & P)	C	N	_____
Urine culture and sensitivity (C & S)	C	N	_____
Sputum for acid fast bacilli (AFB)	C	N	_____
Other _____	C	N	_____

Serology

Human immunodeficiency virus screen (HIVB$_{24}$AG)   C   N   _____

Carcinoembryonic antigen (CEA)   C   N   _____

Rheumatoid Factor (RA)   C   N   _____

Other _____   C   N   _____

Blood Bank

Type and crossmatch (T & X match)   C   N   _____

Packed cells (PC)   C   N   _____

Platelets (plts or plt ct)   C   N   _____

Coombs test   C   N   _____

Other _____   C   N   _____

Cytology

PAP smear   C   N   _____

Other _____   C   N   _____

Other specimens

UA   C   N   _____

CSF   C   N   _____

Bone marrow biopsy   C   N   _____

Pleural fluid   C   N   _____

Other _____   C   N   _____

Point of Care Testing (POCT)

Blood glucose monitoring   C   N   _____

Guaiac all stools   C   N   _____

Other _____   C   N   _____

Objective 6: Transcribe Diagnostic Imaging Orders.

X-ray orders that require preparation

Upper gastrointestinal (UGI)   C   N   _____

Barium enema (BE)   C   N   _____

Intravenous urogram or pyelogram (IVU or IVP)   C   N   _____

X-ray orders that do not require a preparation

Chest PA & Lat   C   N   _____

Kidney, ureters, and bladder (KUB)	C	N	_____
Skeletal X-ray	C	N	_____
Other _____	C	N	_____

Special Procedures

Angiogram, venogram, or arteriogram	C	N	_____
Other _____	C	N	_____

Computed Tomography (CT)

CT of brain	C	N	_____
Other _____	C	N	_____

Magnetic Resonance Imaging (MRI)

Magnetic resonance imaging of spine (MRI)	C	N	_____
Other _____	C	N	_____

Nuclear Medicine

Bone scan	C	N	_____
Body scan (brain, liver, spleen)	C	N	_____
Thyroid uptake scan	C	N	_____
Stress test using Persantine/thallium, etc.	C	N	_____
Other _____	C	N	_____

Ultrasound

Pelvic ultrasound (US)	C	N	_____
Other _____	**C**	**N**	_____

Objective 7: Transcribe respiratory orders.

Diagnostic Orders

Arterial blood gases (ABG)	C	N	_____
Capillary blood gases (CBG)	C	N	_____
Spirometry	C	N	_____

Treatment Orders

Incentive Spirometry	C	N	_____
Small volume nebulizer (SVN)	C	N	_____
Intermittent positive pressure breathing (IPPB)	C	N	_____
Oxygen (O_2)	C	N	_____
Other _____	C	N	_____

Objective 8: Transcribe cardiovascular diagnostic orders.

Electrocardiogram (EKG or ECG)   C   N   _____

2D-M Mode Echocardiogram   C   N   _____

Stress Test   C   N   _____

Other _____   **C**   **N**   _____

Objective 9: Transcribe neurodiagnostic orders.

Electroencephalogram (EEG)   C   N   _____

Brain stem auditory evoked response (BAER)   C   N   _____

Other _____   C   N   _____

Objective 10: Transcribe physical therapy orders.

Whirlpool   C   N   _____

Crutch training   C   N   _____

Exercises   C   N   _____

Hot packs   C   N   _____

Hyperbaric   C   N   _____

Other _____   C   N   _____

Objective 11: Transcribe occupational therapy orders.

Activities of daily living (ADL) evaluation   C   N   _____

Other _____   C   N   _____

Objective 12: Transcribe miscellaneous orders.

Case management   C   N   _____

Social services   C   N   _____

Consult   C   N   _____

Other _____   C   N   _____

Performance Acceptable   ☐

Additional Practice and Re-evaluation Needed   ☐

Recommendations to Improve Performance: _____

_____

_____

_____

Preceptor's Comments: _____

_____

_____

_____

Instructor's Comments: _____

_____

_____

_____

Student's Comments: _____

_____

_____

_____

UNIT 7

Health Unit Coordinating Procedures

The following activities are designed to help you meet the objectives for this unit. You will need to be evaluated by your preceptor or instructor as you perform the activities. Each activity should be completed with a *C* (competent) score by the end of the clinical session.

Objective 1: Perform admission procedures.	Evaluation		Initials
Greet the patient upon arrival at the nurse's station.	C	N	_____
Inform the patient that you will notify the nurse of his or her arrival.	C	N	_____
Notify the attending physician and/or hospital resident of the patient's admission, and obtain orders.	C	N	_____
Move the patient's name from the admission screen on the computer to the correct bed on the nursing unit.	C	N	_____

Record the patient's admission in the admission, discharge, and transfer sheet and the census board.	C N	_____
Check the patient's signature on the admission service agreement form.	C N	_____

Complete the procedure for the preparation of the chart:

a. Label all the chart forms with the patient's identification labels.	C N	_____
b. Fill in all the needed headings.	C N	_____
c. Place all the forms in the chart behind the proper dividers.	C N	_____
Label the outside of the chart.	C N	_____
Prepare any other labels or identification cards used by your facility.	C N	_____
Place the patient identification labels in the correct place in the patient's chart.	C N	_____
Fill in all the necessary information on the patient's Kardex form or into the computer if Kardex is computerized.	C N	_____
Place the Kardex forms in the proper place in the Kardex folder.	C N	_____
Enter appropriate data required into the computer patient profile screen.	C N	_____
Record the data from the admission nurse's notes on the graphic sheet.	C N	_____
Place the allergy information in all the designated areas or write *NKA*.	C N	_____
Prepare an allergy bracelet with allergies written on it to be placed on the patient's wrist if necessary.	C N	_____
Note code status on front of chart if necessary.	C N	_____
Place red tape stating "name alert" on spine of chart if there is another patient on the unit with same or similar name.	C N	_____
Add the patient's name to the required unit forms.	C N	_____
Transcribe the admission orders according to your hospital's policy.	C N	_____

Objective 2: Perform discharge procedures.

Read the entire order when transcribing the discharge order.	C N	_____
Check for any Rx that may have been left in chart by doctor.	C N	_____
Notify the nurse caring for the patient of the discharge order.	C N	_____
Enter a "pending discharge" with expected departure time into the computer.	C N	_____
Explain the procedure for discharge to the patient and/or the patient's relatives.	C N	_____
Notify other departments that may be giving the patient daily treatments.	C N	_____
Communicate the patient's discharge to the dietary department via computer.	C N	_____
Arrange for clinic appointment if doctor requests it.	C N	_____

Prepare credit slips for medications returned to the pharmacy or equipment and supplies from CSD.	C	N	_____
Notify nursing personnel or transportation service to transport patient to the discharge area.	C	N	_____
Write the patient's name on the admission, discharge, and transfer sheet.	C	N	_____
Delete the patient's name from the unit census board and TPR sheet.	C	N	_____
Notify environmental services to clean the discharged patient's room.	C	N	_____
Prepare the chart for the health records department.	C	N	_____
Check the summary/DRG worksheet for the physician's summation and the patient's final diagnosis.	C	N	_____
Check for the correct patient identification labels on chart forms.	C	N	_____
Shred all chart forms that have been labeled and do not have any documentation on them.	C	N	_____
Check for "old records" or "split chart." Place the split chart in the proper sequence.	C	N	_____
Rearrange the chart forms in discharge sequence per your hospital policy.	C	N	_____
Send the chart of the discharged patient to the health records department along with old records of the patient.	C	N	_____

Objective 3: Perform additional steps for discharge to another facility.

Notify case management or social service of the physician's orders to discharge to another facility. Transportation will usually be arranged by the case manager or social worker.	C	N	_____
Complete the continuing care form or transfer form (top section).	C	N	_____
Photocopy forms as necessary (check hospital policy for procedure).	C	N	_____
Distribute continuing care form and copies as required (place a copy of continuing care form and chart copies in envelope to send with patient).	C	N	_____
Perform routine discharge steps.	C	N	_____

Objective 4: Perform additional steps for discharge home with assistance.

Notify case management or social service.	C	N	_____
Prepare the continuing care form.	C	N	_____
Obtain a release of information from patient.	C	N	_____
Photocopy forms as necessary (check hospital policy for procedure).	C	N	_____
Distribute continuing care form and copies as required.	C	N	_____
Perform routine discharge steps.	C	N	_____

Objective 5: Perform postmortem procedures.

Contact the attending physician, staff physician, or resident when asked by nurse to verify the patient's death.	C	N	_____
Notify the hospital operator of patient's death.	C	N	_____
Prepare any forms that may be needed.	C	N	_____
Notify the mortuary that has been requested by the family (if requested to do so).	C	N	_____
Call the morgue if the body is to be taken for autopsy or is to remain there until mortuary personnel arrives.	C	N	_____
The nurse will gather the deceased's clothing and place it in a paper sack; you may be asked to label it with the patient's name, room number and the date.	C	N	_____
Obtain the mortuary book from the nursing office or have a mortuary form prepared for when the mortuary personnel arrive.	C	N	_____
Notify all doctors who were involved with the patient's care	C	N	_____
Perform routine discharge steps.	C	N	_____

Objective 6: Perform procedures for transfer of patient to another unit within the hospital.

Transcribe order for a transfer.	C	N	_____
Notify the nurse caring for the patient of the transfer order.	C	N	_____
Notify admitting department of transfer order to get a room assignment.	C	N	_____
Communicate to the nurse caring for the patient the receiving unit and room number as given by the admitting department.	C	N	_____
Notify the receiving unit of the transfer.	C	N	_____
Record the transfer on the unit admission, discharge, transfer sheet.	C	N	_____
Just before the transfer of the patient, remove the chart forms from the chart holder and the Kardex form from the Kardex holder and obtain any medication administration records not filed in the chart.	C	N	_____
Erase patient's name on the census board.	C	N	_____
Notify all departments that perform regularly scheduled treatments on the patient.	C	N	_____
Indicate the transfer on the computer diet screen and on the TPR sheet.	C	N	_____
Notify the attending physician, all other physicians involved with the patient's care, the switchboard, information desk, the flower desk, and the mail room of the transfer.	C	N	_____
Follow procedures per discharge.	C	N	_____

Objective 7: Perform procedures for transfer of patient to another room on the same unit.

Transcribe order for a transfer. C N _____

Notify the nurse caring for the patient when request for transfer is granted. C N _____

Remove patient's chart from chart holder and place it in chart holder with the new room number after printing corrected ID labels. C N _____

Place all Kardex forms in their new places in the Kardex form holder. C N _____

Move patient's name to the correct bed on computer census screen. C N _____

Send change by computer to the dietary department and change room number on the TPR sheet. C N _____

Record the transfer on the unit admission, discharge, and transfer sheet and on the census board. C N _____

Notify environmental services to clean the room. C N _____

Notify the switchboard and the information center of the change. C N _____

Objective 8: Perform procedures for receiving a transferred patient.

Notify the nurse caring for the patient of the expected arrival of a transferred patient. C N _____

Introduce yourself to the transferred patient upon his or her arrival on the unit. C N _____

Notify the nurse caring for the patient of the transferred patient's arrival. C N _____

Place the patient's chart in the correct chart holder. C N _____

Print corrected patient ID labels and label patient's chart. C N _____

Place allergy label on front of chart if necessary. C N _____

Place all Kardex forms in their proper places. C N _____

Note the receiving of a transfer patient on the unit admission, discharge, and transfer sheet and write the patient's name on the census board. C N _____

Place the patient's name on the TPR sheet. C N _____

Move the patient's name from the unit patient came from and place in correct bed on the computer census screen. C N _____

Transcribe any new doctors' orders. C N _____

Objective 9: Perform preoperative procedures.

Label the surgery forms with the patient's identification labels and place them within the patient's chart. C N _____

Check the patient's chart for the history and physical report. C N _____

Check the patient's chart for the following signed consent forms:

Surgical consent.	C	N	_____
Blood transfusion consent or refusal form.	C	N	_____
Admission service agreement.	C	N	_____

Check the patient's chart for any previously ordered studies such as labs and x-rays.   C   N   _____

Chart the patient's latest vital signs.   C   N   _____

File the current medication administration record in the patient's chart.   C   N   _____

Print at least five face sheets to place in chart.   C   N   _____

Place at least three sheets of patient identification labels in the patient's chart.   C   N   _____

Notify the appropriate nursing personnel when surgery calls for the patient.   C   N   _____

Objective 10: Perform postoperative procedures

Inform the patient's nurse of the patient's arrival in the PACU.   C   N   _____

Inform the patient's nurse of the expected arrival of the patient from the recovery room.   C   N   _____

Place all operating records behind the proper divider.   C   N   _____

Write the date of surgery and the surgical procedure in the designated place on the patient's Kardex form or on the computer.   C   N   _____

Fill in the date of the surgery on the patient's graphic sheet.   C   N   _____

Transcribe the physicians' postoperative orders. Notify the nurse caring for the patient of stat physicians' orders.   C   N   _____

Performance Acceptable   ☐

Additional Practice and Re-evaluation Needed   ☐

Recommendations to Improve Performance: _____

_____

_____

_____

Preceptor's Comments: _____

_____

_____

_____

Instructor's Comments: _____

_____

_____

_____

Student's Comments: _____

_____

_____

_____

UNIT 8

Organization and Prioritizing Skills

The following activities are designed to help you meet the objectives for this unit. You will need to be evaluated by your preceptor or instructor as you perform the activities. Each activity should be completed with a C (competent) score by the end of the clinical session.

Objective 1: Demonstrate knowledge of code procedures.	**Evaluation**		**Initials**
Demonstrate how you would call a code arrest when requested to do so.	C	N	_____
Demonstrate how you would respond to a fire drill when requested to do so.	C	N	_____
Describe your role in case of a disaster code as outlined in the hospital disaster manual.	C	N	_____

Objective 2: Perform tasks in a conscientious manner.

Upon completion of transcription of a set of doctors' orders, ask your preceptor or instructor to evaluate your correct use of symbols.	C	N	_____
Take laboratory test results over the phone. Record the patient's name, room number, the laboratory values, and the date, time, and the caller's name. Read this information back to the caller to check for accuracy.	C	N	_____
When answering the telephone, record in writing any information that must be transferred to another person on the unit.	C	N	_____

Objective 3: Demonstrate accuracy when transcribing doctors' orders.

Before taking transcribed orders to your preceptor for evaluation, check yourself on each of the following. Did you:

Read all of the orders?	C	N	_____

Fax the pharmacy copy?	C	N	_____
Check for stats?	C	N	_____
Notify appropriate person or department of stat orders?	C	N	_____
Place the telephone calls, if necessary?	C	N	_____
Order everything required?	C	N	_____
Kardex all of the orders?	C	N	_____
Communicate the necessary orders to the nursing staff?	C	N	_____
Use correct symbols?	C	N	_____
Sign off the completed orders?	C	N	_____

Your preceptor or instructor will evaluate you on the following:

Charted vital signs without error.	C	N	_____
Labeled chart forms correctly.	C	N	_____
Recorded telephone laboratory values without error.	C	N	_____
Ordered diagnostic tests, treatments, and/or equipment correctly.	C	N	_____

Objective 4: Demonstrate initiative.

Do you participate in planning the daily activities with your preceptor?	C	N	_____
Do you express a desire to perform new and varied skills?	C	N	_____
Do you answer the telephone as quickly as possible?	C	N	_____
Do you use resource material to assist in seeking needed information?	C	N	_____
Do you find something to do when your preceptor is not on the unit?	C	N	_____
Do you take notes so that you can remember what you learned?	C	N	_____

Objective 5: Demonstrate thoroughness.

Check all charts for new doctors' orders before returning the chart to the chart rack.	C	N	_____
Determine to whom a given phone message is to be transferred, rather than giving it to the first possible person.	C	N	_____
Keep a personal record of unfinished tasks you intend to complete as soon as possible.	C	N	_____

Objective 6: Demonstrate ability to establish priorities on the job.

You have returned to the nursing unit from a coffee break. There are several charts in the rack that are flagged to indicate new doctors' orders. Describe how you would proceed with this situation.	C	N	_____
Explain why you should answer a ringing phone before responding to a verbal request if they occur simultaneously, unless it is an emergency situation.	C	N	_____

Explain why a request to take a patient to surgery has more urgency than a request to take a patient to radiology.   C   N   _____

Explain why it is sound management to check the charts of the patients scheduled for surgery that day when you first arrive for duty on the nursing unit.   C   N   _____

Objective 7: Demonstrate ability to multitask.

Handle interruption of telephone calls while transcribing doctors orders.   C   N   _____

Complete routine tasks with interruptions of assisting visitors, doctors, nurses, and others.   C   N   _____

Objective 8: Demonstrate the ability to plan a day's activities.

1. List below the daily routine tasks you are now performing as part of your responsibilities in the nursing unit   C   N   _____

Health Unit Coordinator Tasks

_____

_____

_____

_____

_____

_____

_____

_____

_____

_____

_____

2. Using your task list, plan your work routine for one day.   C   N   _____

Time	**Health Unit Coordinator Tasks**
_____	_____
_____	_____
_____	_____
_____	_____
_____	_____
_____	_____
_____	_____
_____	_____
_____	_____
_____	_____

3. Implement your work schedule plan. Make adjustments as necessary. Critique your plan.   C   N   _____

a. What were the strengths in your plan?

_____

_____

_____

b. What were the weaknesses in your plan?

_____

_____

_____

c. What changes will you make?

_____

_____

_____

Performance Acceptable ☐

Additional Practice and Re-evaluation Needed ☐

Recommendations to Improve Performance: _____

_____

_____

_____

Preceptor's Comments: _____

_____

_____

_____

Instructor's Comments: _____

_____

_____

_____

Student's Comments: _____

_____

_____

_____